D0765794

TO BE RENEWED/RETURNED
ON OR BEFORE THE DATE MARKED BELOW

PLEASE ENTER DETAILS BELOW ON LOAN SLIP

Author

Title

WHJ-0169

Physical Illness and Schizophrenia

A Review of the Evidence

Stefan Leucht

Assistant Professor
Department of Psychiatry and Psychotherapy, Technische Universität München, Germany

Tonja Burkard

Medical Doctor

John H Henderson

Retired Consultant Psychiatrist

Mario Maj

Professor of Psychiatry and Chairman of the Department of Psychiatry, University of Naples, Italy

Norman Sartorius

President, International Association for the Improvement of Mental Health Programmes
Adjunct Professor of Psychiatry, Washington University, USA
Professor of Psychiatry, University of Zagreb
Visiting Professor of Psychiatry, Universities of Beijing, London and Prague

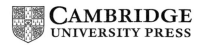
CAMBRIDGE
UNIVERSITY PRESS

CAMBRIDGE UNIVERSITY PRESS
Cambridge, New York, Melbourne, Madrid, Cape Town, Singapore, São Paulo

Cambridge University Press
The Edinburgh Building, Cambridge CB2 8RU, UK

Published in the United States of America by Cambridge University Press, New York

www.cambridge.org
Information on this title: www.cambridge.org/9780521882644

© Cambridge University Press 2007

First published 2007

Printed in the United Kingdom at the University Press, Cambridge

A catalogue record for this publication is available from the British Library

ISBN-978-0-521-88264-4 paperback

Contents

Preface

This is the first of a series of volumes addressing an issue which is emerging as a priority in the mental health field: the timely and proper recognition of physical health problems in people with severe mental disorders.

It is now well documented by research that people with severe mental disorders have a higher prevalence of several physical diseases and a higher mortality from natural causes than the general population. They seem not to have benefited from the recent favourable trends concerning mortality due to some physical diseases, in particular cardiovascular illness. Their access to physical healthcare is reduced and the quality of the physical care they receive is worse as compared with the general population. If we are really concerned about the quality of life of people with mental disorders and wish to protect their civil rights, we cannot ignore the fact that physical health is a crucial dimension of their quality of life, and that access to a physical healthcare of the same quality as that available to the rest of the population is one of their basic rights as human beings and as citizens.

The initial trigger for the preparation of this series of books has been a personal communication to one of us from a physician working with the Médecins sans Frontières in a Central Asian republic. He felt desperate because he was unable to get sufficient resources to deal with the very high mortality of people with schizophrenia admitted to the central mental hospital in the country: according to his account, one person out of two admitted for schizophrenia was likely to be dead at the end of the year in which he/she was admitted for treatment. Some of the excess mortality would be due, like in other countries, to suicide, but a large proportion of those who would die would have a physical disease (e.g. tuberculosis) as the main cause of death.

Indeed, mental hospitals in many countries are often lacking equipment that could help in making the diagnosis of physical illness as well as medications and other material that would make it possible to recognize and treat physical illness. Psychiatrists are reluctant to treat physical illness, perhaps as frequently as doctors in other medical specialties fail to recognize that their patients also suffer from a mental disorder or refuse to provide treatment for it.

Why people with mental illness are more likely to have a physical illness than the rest of the population is only partially known. Part of the answer to this question may be that some people with mental illness do not pay sufficient attention to their bodies and do not follow elementary rules of hygiene and disease prophylaxis. The fact that they often live in conditions of poverty and are exposed to considerable dangers of violence and abuse might also explain some of the excess morbidity and mortality from physical illness that they have. The fact that people with mental illness may be abusing alcohol or taking drugs and that they are therefore exposed to the health consequences of substance abuse and diseases related to the manner of use of drugs (e.g. hepatitis) may also play a role. There remains, however, a substantial proportion of excess physical morbidity that is not explicable by the above-mentioned factors, and it is therefore necessary to suppose that there are factors that facilitate the occurrence of physical illness and are inherent in people who have mental disorders. Changes in the immune system and hormonal imbalance have been mentioned as being among those factors, but it is obvious that more research will be necessary to unravel the puzzle of high rates of physical illness in people with mental disorders.

In many countries psychiatrists have taken off their white coats, shed the symbols of being physicians, forgetting that they are medical doctors – with a particular interest in mental symptoms but still essentially practitioners of a medical discipline. The creation of the specialty of liaison psychiatry is a sad testimony to the fact that only a small proportion of psychiatrists have an interest in dealing in a comprehensive manner with people struck by illness. There are no liaison internists, liaison dermatologists nor liaison surgeons: when invited to consult other colleagues, they simply do that without creating a subgroup that will be specially trained to do this. The existence of liaison psychiatrists is an unwise message to the rest of medicine: despite having a medical diploma, only a few among the psychiatrists are sufficiently well trained in medicine to be able to deal with patients who have a mental and a physical disease at the same time.

What should be done about this? The first step is raising awareness of the problem among mental healthcare professionals, primary care providers, patients with mental illness and their families. Education and training of mental health professionals and primary care providers is a further essential step. Mental health professionals should be trained to perform at least basic medical tasks. They should be educated about the importance of recognizing physical illness in people with severe mental disorders, and encouraged to familiarize themselves with the most common reasons for underdiagnosis or misdiagnosis of physical illness in these people. On the other hand, primary care providers should overcome their reluctance to treat people with severe mental illness, and learn effective ways to interact and communicate with them: it is not only an issue of knowledge and skills, but most of all one of attitudes.

Another essential step is the development of an appropriate integration between mental health and physical healthcare. There is some debate in the literature about who should monitor physical health in people with severe mental disorders. However, the crucial point is that there should always be 'somebody' in charge of this problem (i.e. a well-identified professional should be responsible for the physical healthcare of each patient).

Finally, further research in this area is needed. Physical illnesses should not be always regarded as confounding variables in studies dealing with mental illness. Physical comorbidity should be studied systematically, so that the interaction between the various mental disorders and the different physical diseases – in inpatients as well as in outpatients, in women as well as in men, and in young people as well as in the elderly – can be better understood.

This series of books aims to contribute to several of the above steps, by providing a comprehensive review of current research evidence on the prevalence of the various physical diseases in people with the most common mental disorders, and by identifying possible targets for future research. We hope the volume will be useful not only to policy-makers and mental health professionals, but also to primary care practitioners and at least to some extent to those who receive care from mental health services and their families.

Acknowledgements

We wish to thank Professors and Doctors A. de Leon, A. H. Friedlander, D. Lawrence, K. Hatta, D. Lawrence, K. Hatta, D. Templer, R. McCreadie, D. Perkins, P. B. Mortensen, J. K. Rybakowski, I. Steiner, M. U. Mondelli, R. Oken, J. Newcomer and F. Cournos for reviewing parts of this review. Evelyn Dass is thanked for her help with the literature search and the Association for the Improvement of Mental Health Programmes for its support. Eli Lilly provided an unrestricted educational grant to the latter association.

Thanks to John Langerholc for his correction of the draft.

Abbreviations

AD	Alzheimer's disease
ADH	antidiuretic hormone
AHA	American Heart Association
AIDS	acquired immundeficiency syndrome
AMI	acute myocardial infarction
AML	amyotrophic lateral sclerosis
AP	angina pectoris
ARA	American Rheumatism Association
ASA	arylsulphatase A
ASA-CS	arylsulphatase A cerebroside sulphate
ASA-NCS	arylsulphatase A nitrocatechol sulphate
ATP	Adult Treatment Panel (definition of metabolic syndrome)
BDV	Borna disease virus
BMC	bone mineral content
BMD	bone mineral density
BMI	body mass index
CATIE	Clinical Trials of Antipsychotic Treatment Effectiveness
CI	confidence internal
CNS	central nervous system
COPD	chronic obstructive pulmonary disease
CPK	creatinine phosphokinase
CSF	cerebrospinal fluid
D2	dopamine 2
DEXA	dual-energy X-ray absorptiometry
DM	diabetes mellitus
DMFT	decayed, missing and filled teeth
DNA	deoxyribonucleic acid
DSM-III	Diagnostic and Statistical Manual of Mental Disorders, 3rd revision
DSM-IV	Diagnostic and Statistical Manual of Mental Disorders, 4th revision
ECG	electrocardiogram
EEG	electroencephalogram

EFT_4	estimated free thyroxine
ESR	erythrocyte sedimentation rate
EPS	extrapyramidal side-effects/symptoms
ESS	euthyroid sick syndrome
FEV_1	forced expiratory volume
FSH	follicle-stimulating hormone
FT_3I	free triiodothyronine index
FT_4I	free thyroxine index
FVC	forced vital capacity
GBV-C	GB virus-C (GB, initials of the first patient)
GRH	gonadotropin-releasing hormone
HBV	hepatitis B virus
HbsAg	hepatitis B surface antigen
HCV	hepatitis C virus
HDL	high-density lipoprotein
HDL-C	high-density lipoprotein cholesterol
HGV	hepatitis G virus
HIV	human immunodeficiency virus
HTLV-1	human T-cell lymphotrophic virus type 1
IBS	irritable bowel syndrome
ICD-10	International Classification of Diseases, 10th revision
IFG	impaired fasting glucose
IgE	immunoglobulin E
IGT	impaired glucose tolerance
IHD	ischaemic heart disease
IRR	incidence rate ratio
i.v.	intravenous
LDL	low-density lipoprotein
LH	luteinizing hormone
MEDLINE	Online database of 11 million citations and abstracts from health and medical journals and other news sources
MI	myocardial infarction
MeSH	Medical Subject Headings
MLD	metachromatic leukodystrophy
MS	metabolic syndrome
n	number
NAD	nicotinamide/ nicotine acid
NDWG	normalized diurnal weight gain
n.s.	not statistically significant
NTI	non-thyroidal illness
OR	odds ratio
OSA	obstructive sleep apnoea
p	significance level

PBCs	pregnancy and birth complications
PCR	polymerase chain reaction
PD	polydipsia
PU	polyuria
QTc	rate-corrected QT interval
RA	rheumatoid arthritis
RateR	rate ratio
RR	relative risk
RRBP	Riva Rocci/blood pressure
s.	statistically significant
SAD	schizoaffective disorder
SIDS	sudden infant death syndrome
SIR	standardized incidence rate
SMR	standardized morbidity ratio
SPGU	specific gravity of urine
STEP	Schizophrenia Treatment and Education Program
T_3	triiodothyronine
T_4	thyroxine
TBE	tick-borne encephalitis
TBG	thyroxine-finding globulin
TCI	transient cerebral ischaemia
TMD	temporomandibular disorder
TRH	thyrotropin-releasing hormone
TSH	thyroid-stimulating hormone
TTV	TT-virus (TT, initials of the first patient)
URI	upper respiratory infections
VA	ventricular arrhythmia
WI	water intoxication

Introduction

Schizophrenia is a chronic disease that afflicts approximately 1% of the population worldwide (Freedman 2003). It usually afflicts people at a young age and, according to a report of the World Health Organization, it is among the seven most disabling diseases in the age group between 20 and 45, far surpassing diabetes, HIV or cardiovascular diseases (World Health Organization 2001). A number of reviews have shown that there is an excess mortality in people with schizophrenia, the overall mortality being twice as high as that in the general population (Allebeck 1989, Brown 1997, Colton and Manderscheid 2006, Harris and Barraclough 1998), so that schizophrenia has been called a 'life-shortening disease'(Allebeck 1989). Suicide and accidents account for about 40% of this excess mortality (Baxter and Appleby 1999, Black *et al.* 1985, Palmer *et al.* 2005, Tsuang *et al.* 1999); the rest is due to physical illness. Despite this excess mortality due to physical diseases, the concern for the somatic well-being of people with schizophrenia has been neglected for decades. A number of reasons account for this neglect, one of them being the stigma related to psychiatric disorders (Sartorius and Schulze 2005). A recent population-wide study in Australia (Lawrence *et al.* 2003) showed that although people with schizophrenia suffer more frequently from cardiovascular problems than the general population, they receive revascularization procedures less frequently than the general population. People with mental disorders were also reported to be less likely to be placed on HbA1c and cholesterol monitoring (Jones *et al.* 2004), to have a retinal examination if they have diabetes (Desai *et al.* 2002), to be treated for osteoporosis (Bishop *et al.* 2004) or to receive medical visits (Cradock-O'Leary *et al.* 2002, Folsom *et al.* 2002); and they are treated for a physical disease only if it is life-threatening (Munck-Jorgensen *et al.* 2000).

While the excess mortality of people with schizophrenia has been well established (Allebeck 1989, Brown 1997, Harris and Barraclough 1998), no comprehensive review of the comorbidity of schizophrenia with physical illness is available to date. Such data would be useful, because a review of the excess rates of *comorbidities* rather than excess *mortality* assesses the problem at a stage when interventions are still possible. The main aim of this book was to fill this gap by providing a comprehensive review of the epidemiological literature on the association between schizophrenia and comorbid medical illnesses. Hypotheses explaining excess or reduced rates are also listed. The review may thus serve as a basis for projects for improving the physical health of people with schizophrenia.

Method

A search in MEDLINE (1966 – last update May 2006) was made to find epidemiological studies on the association between schizophrenia and physical illnesses. A broad search strategy had to be used to ensure that no physical illness had been missed. For this reason the MeSH term for schizophrenia was combined with the 23 MeSH terms for the general disease categories of physical diseases. If the search had been performed for each individual physical disease alone, some diseases could have easily been missed. These MeSH terms were:

- Bacterial Infections and Mycoses
- Virus Diseases (+ HIV)
- Parasitic Diseases
- Neoplasms
- Musculoskeletal Diseases
- Digestive System Diseases
- Stomatognathic Diseases
- Respiratory Tract Diseases
- Otorhinolaryngologic Diseases
- Diseases of the Nervous System: autoimmune diseases of the nervous system, autonomic nervous system diseases, central nervous system diseases *(brain diseases, CNS infections, encephalomyelitis, high-pressure neurological syndrome, meningitis, movement disorders, ocular motility disorders, pneumocephalus, spinal cord diseases)*, chronobiology disorders, cranial nerve diseases, demyelinating diseases, nervous system malformations, nervous system neoplasms, neurocutaneous syndrome, neurodegenerative diseases, neurologic manifestations, neuromuscular diseases, neurotoxicity syndromes, sleep disorders, trauma, nervous system
- Eye Diseases
- Urologic and Male Genital Diseases
- Female Genital Diseases and Pregnancy Complications
- Cardiovascular Diseases
- Hemic and Lymphatic Diseases

- Congenital, Hereditary and Neonatal Diseases and Abnormalities
- Skin and Connective Tissue Diseases
- Nutritional and Metabolic Diseases
- Endocrine Diseases
- Immune System Diseases
- Disorders of Environmental Origin
- Animal diseases
- Pathological Conditions, Signs and Symptoms.

All abstracts found were read, and potentially relevant articles were ordered for more detailed inspection. The first search was made in autumn 2004; an update search was made in May 2006. The search was complemented by relevant articles mentioned in the studies and other reviews identified. In addition, the drafts of each thematic chapter were sent to experts with the request for information on studies that were missed by our search (see Acknowledgements).

At the beginning of each section we indicate how many references were found by the MEDLINE search and how many references were added from other sources (mainly cross-referencing). These numbers relate solely to the epidemiological studies included in the various sections, not to references for e.g. definitions, hypotheses etc. The aim of this description was to provide some information about the search and on how many studies were found for each category.

There was no restriction as to language.

The focus was on comorbidity studies rather than on mortality studies, since, on the one hand, mortality studies had already been well summarized in other reviews (Allebeck 1989, Brown 1997, Harris and Barraclough 1998). Furthermore, the interest in doing a review of comorbidity studies lies in these studies which assess the associations at a stage when interventions are still possible. Studies that were concerned with mere side-effects of antipsychotic drugs rather than true comorbid diseases were also excluded. Sometimes, however, this distinction was difficult. For example, weight gain is a side-effect of antipsychotic drugs, but the resulting obesity and its potential consequences are major health problems.

Given that the general quality of the studies identified varied substantially from one disease category to another, it was not possible to apply the same inclusion and exclusion criteria for all disease categories. For example, while there are many high-quality, population-based studies on the association between schizophrenia and cancer, the literature on bacterial infections in schizophrenia is much more limited. The aim of the review was not only to find out for which areas compelling evidence is already available, but also whether according to preliminary evidence there are areas of potential importance that could be the focus of future research. Therefore the inclusion criteria such as e.g. 'only population-based studies' or 'only controlled studies' could not be applied to all chapters. Rather, in well-researched areas (such as that of comorbidity of cancer and schizophrenia), we included only the high-quality studies (in particular, population-based studies with a control group), whereas in areas where only very few studies were available, studies of lower quality such as case series were also included.

When the same study was found several times in different searches, it was described only once in the best fitting category. On the other hand, some studies examined more than one comorbid condition. They were then reported in different chapters. Due to the heterogeneity in terms of quality and designs, meta-analytic calculations were not possible, but rather the results were described in a narrative way. Potential explanations for increased or decreased rates of some physical illnesses are also summarized. Finally, informations on the country of origin of the studies are presented, so as to address the question of whether the results can be generalized to all patients with schizophrenia or are limited only to specific populations.

Results

Figure 3.1 shows the results of the MEDLINE search for the different MeSH terms. It yielded the greatest number of hits on *Diseases of the Nervous System*, followed by *Pathologic Signs and Conditions* and *Disorders of Environmental Origin*, but the latter two were supplemental categories that provided only few new data (see below). The following text addresses the results in the same sequence in which the MeSH terms are listed in MEDLINE.

3.1. Bacterial infections and mycoses

The MEDLINE search on *Bacterial Infections and Mycoses* yielded 277 hits. None of the reports was relevant. Five reports were added from other MEDLINE searches.

3.1.1. *Borrelia burgdorferi*

Brown (1996) identified geographical distributions of bacterial infections and schizophrenia. He found that areas in the United States with high rates of tick-borne encephalitis (TBE) correlated significantly with areas with high schizophrenia rates. He described a similar distribution and correlation in European countries (Croatia, Norway, Finland, Germany, Ireland and others). However, this was only a hypothesis-generating study with a line stating that 'the opinion expressed in the article are solely those of the author...'. Brown also concluded that definite proof of an association could not be demonstrated because of incomplete epidemiological data.

3.1.2. Tuberculosis

Ohta *et al.* (1988) investigated the incidence of tuberculosis among 3251 Japanese patients with a diagnosis of schizophrenia. The incidence of

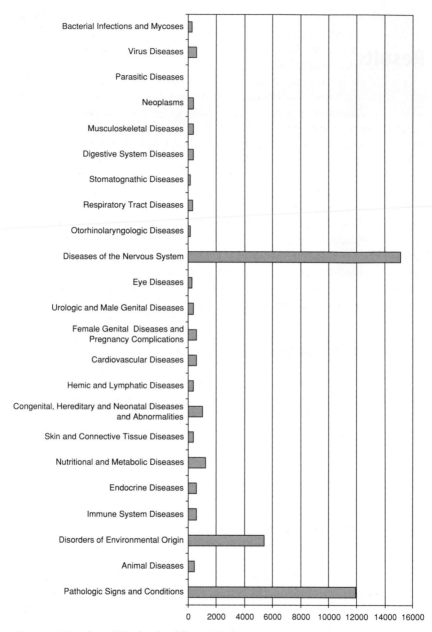

Figure 3.1 Number of hits for the different MeSH terms.

tuberculosis was significantly higher (3.04) in schizophrenic patients than in the general population. In addition to some mortality studies they quoted only the Oxford Record Linkage Study (Baldwin 1979), which also found an increased rate of tuberculosis in schizophrenia.

Fisher *et al.* (1996) examined 113 patients with severe mental illness for tuberculosis. Active respiratory tuberculosis were found in 4.4% of the cases, foci of indefinite activity were found in 3.5% and post-tubercular changes in the lungs and the pleura were found in 7.1% of the cases.

Zeenreich *et al.* (1998) found a prevalence of 5.4% cases of active pulmonary tuberculosis in 720 hospitalized patients during the period 1983–96 in Israel. There was no control group. Zeenreich and colleagues recommended routine screening of all new patients and control screenings to determine if there were cases of tuberculosis to prevent recurrent outbreaks of tuberculosis.

Lawrence *et al.* (2001) observed 3368 schizophrenic male patients and 1674 female schizophrenic patients in Western Australia from 1980 to 1998. They found a first-time hospitalization rate ratio for tuberculosis of 3.04 (n.s.) in male patients and of 2.26 (s.) in female patients.

In summary, it appears that the association between bacterial infections, mycoses and schizophrenia has been insufficiently studied in comorbidity studies. The only bacterial infection for which some evidence is available is tuberculosis. This contrasts with mortality studies in which increased rates of excess mortality due to infections has been demonstrated (Harris and Barraclough 1998). Alternative explanations are that the evidence is buried in old studies that can not be detected by MEDLINE (which starts in 1966), but the older studies would no longer necessarily be representative. Since in some countries, such as Romania, specific wards for people with both schizophrenia and tuberculosis exist, further analyses of these preventable causes of death are warranted.

3.2. Virus diseases

The MEDLINE search on *Virus Diseases* yielded 448 hits. Given the importance of the association between schizophrenia and HIV another MEDLINE search for *HIV* was added which yielded another 153 hits. A total of 62 reports were ordered, of which 14 were included; and 35 reports were added by cross-referencing. Many of the reports investigated the 'viral hypothesis' of schizophrenia, i.e. the question whether virus infections play an aetiological role in the development of schizophrenia, which is not within the scope of this review. Only the studies on HIV and hepatitis were related to physical comorbidity.

3.2.1. Influenza virus

Probably the best-studied association is that of maternal infection with the influenza virus during pregnancy as a risk factor for the later development of schizophrenia. Since by definition these studies considered the rates of influenza infection in mothers of people with schizophrenia rather than examining the prevalence of influenza in schizophrenia, these studies were excluded a priori. Nevertheless, a review on the topic has been provided by Ebert and Kotler (2005), in which 11 out of 19 studies showed a significant relationship between exposure to influenza virus in mid-pregnancy (second trimester) whereas eight did not. The authors concluded that the relationship between influenza virus and schizophrenia is still incompletely understood.

Lawrence et al. (2001) analysed 3368 schizophrenic male patients and 1674 female schizophrenic patients in Western Australia. They found a first-time hospitalization rate ratio for influenza of 1.35 (n.s.) in males and of 0.27 (s.) in females compared to the general population.

3.2.2. Herpes simplex type 1 and 2, rubella virus, measles virus, cytomegalovirus, Epstein–Barr virus

Halone et al. (1974) found increased rates of herpes simplex type 1 antibodies in 54 patients with schizophrenia, although the rates were higher in patients with psychotic depression. No differences in rubella virus titres compared to medical personnel were found, and measles virus titres were even slightly lower among the psychiatric patients.

Rimon et al. (1979) measured immunoglobulin G antibodies to herpes simplex type 1 virus in 16 patients with schizophrenia and found no significant differences in the antibody levels between the schizophrenic patients and normal controls.

Delisi et al. (1986) did not find significantly higher herpes simplex and cytomegalovirus titres in schizophrenics; Epstein–Barr virus titres were increased though not only in patients with schizophrenia but also in non-ill siblings and hospital staff.

Conejero-Goldberg et al. (2003) screened post-mortem orbital frontal brain samples from patients with schizophrenia and compared them with healthy controls. They found no evidence of herpesvirus DNA in the 24 psychiatric cases and the 25 normal controls. Other studies on the prevalence of herpes simplex type 1 antibodies in patients with schizophrenia have been mentioned. It seems that the results were conflicting, i.e. while several studies found increased levels of herpes simplex antibodies in schizophrenic patients, others found no differences between schizophrenics and controls.

3.2.3. Human T-cell lymphotropic virus type 1

Based on previous studies which reported an 18-fold higher incidence of schizophrenia among second-generation Afro-Caribbeans, especially in Jamaican males (Harrison et al. 1988, Harvey et al. 1990), Rodgers-Johnson et al.

(1996) were interested in the role of a novel virus as an aetiological agent for schizophrenia. They examined the retrovirus human T-cell lymphotropic virus type 1 (HTLV-1) as a possibility; because HTLV-1 is endemic in the Caribbean, it is known to be neuropathogenic and can be transmitted perinatally, by sexual contact, blood transfusion and intravenous drug abuse. The prevalence of HTLV-1 infection in 201 Afro-Caribbean psychiatric inpatients was compared with rates in a control hospital population and rates in the healthy Jamaican population. The prevalence was 10% in psychiatric patients and 7% in the control hospital population; the prevalence in the Jamaican population ranged from 1.7% to 17.4% depending on age, gender and social class. The results did not support an aetiological relationship between HTLV-1 and schizophrenia.

3.2.4. Borna disease virus

Taieb *et al.* (2001) reviewed 17 studies using serologic tests or polymerase chain reaction to detect Borna disease virus (BDV) in psychiatric patients. Most studies have sought BDV infection markers in patients with schizophrenia and mood disorders, but BDV may also be involved in other disorders such as autism. The reviewed data supported the assumption that BDV can infect humans and persist in the CNS. While some studies showed an increased prevalence of BDV in psychiatric samples, the contribution of BDV to the physiopathology of mental disorders is not proven by this association. They concluded that further research on the association of schizophrenia and Borna disease virus is warranted.

3.2.5. Human immunodeficiency virus

The association between serious mental illness and human immunodeficiency virus (HIV) serum positivity is well studied. A number of reviews on the prevalence of HIV in mental disorders are available (Cournos and McKinnon 1997, Gottesman and Groome 1997, Grassi 1996, Sewell 1996). Table 3.1 summarizes the results of these reviews as supplemented by further trials identified by our search. The prevalence of HIV among people with serious mental disorders varied quite substantially within a range of 1.30% to 22.9%. In contrast, the latest reported prevalence estimation of HIV in the general population of North America was 0.4% (World Health Organization 2004).

Although evidence clearly shows that rates of HIV infection are increased in schizophrenia, a number of methodological issues require a comment. A first problem is that many studies considered psychiatric patients in general so that those with a primary diagnosis of intravenous substance abuse were not excluded and may have increased the perceived risk. Almost no study exclusively examined the prevalence of HIV in schizophrenia. However, after schizophrenia has been differentiated from rates among other psychotic disorders, no significant differences emerge (Wainberg *et al.* 2003).

Table 3.1. Prevalence of HIV in patients with mental disorders

Reference	Country	Number of patients (n), various psychiatric diagnoses	Number of patients with schizophrenia (%)	HIV positive (% of total sample)
Zamperetti et al. 1990[a]	Italy	475	n.i.	6.5
Sacks et al. 1990[a]	USA	205	25.0	7.8
Cournos et al. 1991[a]	USA	451	65.4	5.5
Volavka et al. 1991	USA	515	74.9	8.9
Lee et al. 1992	USA	135	n.i.	16.3
Sacks et al. 1992	USA	350	n.i.	7.0
Empfield et al. 1993	USA	209	97.0	6.4
Meyer et al. 1993	USA	199	70.4	4.0
Susser et al. 1993	USA	90	65.5	19.0
Chen 1994	Taiwan	834	n.i.	0.0
Cournos et al. 1994	USA	971	n.i.	5.2 (men), 5.3 (women)
Dasananjali 1994	Thailand	325	78.0	1.8
Naber et al. 1994	Germany	623	n.i.	4.8
Silberstein et al. 1994	USA	118	n.i.	22.9
Stewart et al. 1994	USA	533	40.5	5.8
Schwartz-Watts et al. 1995	USA	223	n.i.	5.4
Ayuso-Mateos et al. 1997	Spain	390	n.i.	5.1
Rosenberg et al. 2001	USA	931	n.i.	3.1
Blank et al. 2002	USA	S: 8208, C (Medicaid population): 374 253	100.0	S: 1.2, C: 0.6
Baillargeon et al. 2003	USA	336 668	n.i.	S: 1.30, SAD: 1.67, Non-schizophrenic psychotic disorders: 3.62
Chafetz et al. 2005	USA	781	34.7	S: 4.8, patients with other psychiatric diagnoses: 7.1

[a] Please note that the publications by Zamperetti et al. 1990, Sacks et al. 1990 and Cournos et al. 1991 appear to be preliminary or subgroup reports of later publications.

C, control group; n.i., not indicated; S, patients with schizophrenia; SAD, schizoaffective disorders.

Source: Adapted from Cournos and McKinnon (1997), Gottesman and Groome (1997), Grassi (1996), Sewell (1996) and supplemented by our MEDLINE search.

A second issue is that the vast majority of the studies summarized in Table 3.1 were carried out in the United States, and most of them on the east coast, especially in New York, which is a high-risk area. Studies in Europe (Ayuso-Mateos *et al.* 1997, Naber *et al.* 1994, Zamperetti *et al.* 1990) also showed an increased HIV prevalence rate of about 5%, which contrasts with an estimated prevalence rate <1% in the general European population (World Health Organization 2004), but the rates were not as dramatic as in some of the American studies. In two studies, from Taiwan (Chen 1994) and Thailand (Dasananjali 1994), the prevalence was even lower.

There is a large body of literature on reasons explaining the high HIV prevalence in mentally ill people. There are a number of risk factors. One is the well-known high rate of substance abuse in the mentally ill (Dixon *et al.* 1991, Drake and Wallach 1989, Drake *et al.* 1996, Test *et al.* 1989). Substance abuse is linked to HIV infection, both directly in the case of injecting drug use, and indirectly through its association with unsafe sexual behaviour. There were also a number of studies discussing sexual risk behaviours (multiple and high-risk sex partners, lack of condom use, engaging in same-sex sexual activity, trading sex for money and drugs, coerced sex) that may be more common among psychiatric patients than in the general population (for review see Gottesman and Groome 1997 and Meyer and Nasrallah 2003). These findings contrast in part with a reduced sexual interest in diseases such as schizophrenia, but it has been contended that the sex that mentally ill people are engaged in is riskier from the perspective of acquiring HIV and other sexually transmitted diseases. Another reason for the high prevalence seems to be related to the extent to which a patient with a mental disorder is protected by a country's social security system. For the United States Gottesman and Groome (1997) suggested that deinstitutionalization of the mentally ill (Torrey 1997) is a risk factor, because people with schizophrenia in the community are less able to take care of their health and are not aware of the risk factors for HIV infection. Many people with schizophrenia in the United States are homeless. In contrast, Wainberg *et al.* (2003) suggested that extended periods of institutionalization in same-sex units in hospitals, shelters or prisons may increase high-risk same-sex activity even if the occupants do not identify themselves as gay or lesbian. They recommended that condoms should be available to all patients in psychiatric institutions.

Finally, there are a number of studies on the question of whether mentally ill people have a reduced knowledge about HIV infection risks and AIDS-related issues. In schizophrenia, this question may be especially important due to the cognitive deficits associated with the disorder. Although the results are not fully conclusive (Wainberg *et al.* 2003), appropriate information and educational and preventional programmes have been called for (Gottesman and Groome 1997, Seeman *et al.* 1990, Wainberg *et al.* 2003).

3.2.6. Hepatitis B and C viruses

Hepatitis B and C viruses are transmitted by contact with blood or sexual contact or from mother to infant (Cotran *et al.* 1989). The prevalence of hepatitis B (HBV) in the general population of the United States is estimated to be 4.9% (Rosenberg *et al.* 2001) and that of hepatitis C (HCV) to be 1.8% (Wainberg *et al.* 2003). Since the path of transmission is similar to that of HIV, a higher prevalence was suspected among schizophrenic patients because of their illness-related behaviours. However, much less research on hepatitis in psychiatric disorders is available.

Chaudhury *et al.* (1994) examined 100 institutionalized patients with psychosis and an equal number of age- and sex-matched healthy controls from the same regional background on the prevalence of Australia antigen (HbsAg). The prevalence of HbsAg was 11 to 2, respectively. The authors concluded that institutionalized psychotic patients seem to be at high risk of hepatitis B virus infection.

A Italian study by Cividini *et al.* (1997) investigated 1180 patients with different psychiatric disorders (mental retardation, psychosis and dementia). They found an HCV prevalence of 6.7%. Psychosis and a history of trauma were statistically significant independent risk factors associated with HCV infection. Prolonged residence in psychiatric institutions per se did not entail a significant risk of acquiring HCV infection.

Said *et al.* (2001) investigated the prevalence rate of HBV among schizophrenic patients in Jordan. Hepatitis B is endemic in parts of Asia. The prevalence of hepatitis B surface antigen (HbsAg) among 192 schizophrenic patients was 7.3% while only 2.1% of 192 age- and sex-matched healthy controls tested positive for HbsAg. However, the difference was not statistically significant.

Lawrence *et al.* (2001) screened 3368 schizophrenic male patients and 1674 schizophrenic female patients in Western Australia. They found a first-time hospitalization rate for viral hepatitis of 3.58 (n.s.) in males and 4.93 (n.s.) in females.

Rosenberg *et al.* (2001) found a prevalence of 23.4%/19.6% of HBV/HCV among 931 psychiatric patients from various hospitals on the east coast of the United States.

Nakamura *et al.* (2004) investigated 1193 Japanese psychiatric inpatients (37.6% with schizophrenia, 40.2% psychoactive drug users and 22.2% with various other psychiatric disorders) for the prevalence of HCV. Control data were taken from 197 827 voluntary blood donors from the same prefecture. The prevalence in the schizophrenia group was 6.2% compared with 1.2% in the control group. Mainly older patients (high prevalence in the group over 60 years of age) accounted for the high prevalence in the schizophrenic group.

There exist no studies on knowledge about the path of HCV transmission among psychiatric patients. Clinicians should be aware of the meagre knowledge about HCV among psychiatric patients and should supply appropriate information (Wainberg *et al.* 2003).

In summary, although few studies have been published, the available evidence suggests that rates of HBV infection are increased in schizophrenia.

3.2.7. Hepatitis GB-C/HG and TT viruses

Kalkan *et al.* (2005) investigated 56 schizophrenic patients in Eastern Anatolia, Turkey on the prevalence of the GB virus-C/hepatitis G virus (GBV-C/HGV) and the TT virus (TTV). A total of 26.7% schizophrenic patients tested positive for TTV DNA and 1.7% tested positive for GBV-C/HGV RNA. All patients concerned had a duration of illness longer than 10 years, and the mean institutionalization period was 6.14 ± 1.1 years. Nevertheless the authors concluded that institutionalization and mental or physical disabilities do not constitute an additional risk for TTV infection because they found similar results in other patient groups (mentally retarded children 30.6%, leprosy patients 32.5%, chronic hepatitis B patients 31.3%, hepatitis C patients 53.1% and blood donors 16.8%).

3.3. Parasitic diseases

The MEDLINE search on *Parasitic Diseases* yielded 56 hits. Nine studies were ordered, of which five were relevant.

3.3.1. *Toxoplasma gondii*

Many studies focussed on the association between schizophrenia and *Toxoplasma gondii*. It is important to note from the very beginning that this research has been driven by a hypothesis suggesting that (similar to the virus hypothesis) *Toxoplasma gondii* may be an aetiological factor for the development of schizophrenia rather than a clinically significant comorbid condition. Therefore, in the studies on this question, investigators considered the number of patients with increased *Toxoplasma gondii* antibodies rather than how many patients suffered from clinically manifest infection. In 18 of the 19 studies published between 1953 and 2003 and reviewed by Torrey and Yolken (2003), patients with schizophrenia had increased *Toxoplasma gondii* antibody titers. The difference was statistically significant in 11 studies. Our search identified two further studies that were not included by Torrey and Yolken (2003).

An early study by Destounis (1966) observed higher rates of positive skin tests for toxoplasmosis in schizophrenic patients compared with a non-schizophrenic control group.

Conejero-Goldberg *et al.* (2003), however, screened 51 post-mortem orbital frontal brain samples from patients with schizophrenia, affective disorders and controls for the presence of herpesvirus and *Toxoplasma gondii*. They found no sequences of *Toxoplasma gondii* and only two sequences of HHV-6B (one from a case with bipolar disorder and one from a control).

Toxoplasma gondii is of interest as a possible aetiology of schizophrenia because of its known affinity for brain tissue and its capacity for long-term infection starting in early life (Torrey and Yolken 2003). There is also some evidence suggesting that people with schizophrenia may have been exposed more frequently to cats in childhood. However, the high prevalence of *Toxoplasma gondii* titres may also be due to disease-related differential exposure in the sense that hospitalized patients with schizophrenia may be fed on undercooked meat (Torrey and Yolken 2003). In conclusion, the research on the association between *Toxoplasma gondii* and schizophrenia has been driven by the infectious hypothesis of schizophrenia, and the evidence is inconclusive. Whether *Toxoplasma gondii* is a clinically relevant comorbidity in schizophrenia has not been examined.

3.3.2. Chlamydial infections

Fellerhoff *et al.* (2005) investigated the prevalence of the intracellular parasites Chlamydiaceae. They found a significant prevalence of *Chlamydophila psittaci*, *C. pneumoniae* and *Chlamydia trachomatis* (9/18, 50%), as compared to controls (8/115, 6.97%). The authors reported that treatment with vitro-activated immune cells together with antibiotic modalities showed sustained mental improvements in patients that did not depend on treatment with antipsychotic drugs. They recommended further controlled studies including sham treatment of patients to support their findings.

3.3.3. Intestinal parasitic infections

Cheng and Wang (2005) examined a total of 464 patients from seven psychiatric hospitals in North Taiwan to establish the prevalence of nosocomial infections of intestinal parasites. They found that 8.4% were infected with one or more intestinal parasites. It was surprising that higher positive rates were found among patients with non-schizophrenic diseases (14.1%) than those with schizophrenia (6.8%). The positive rate was significantly higher in males (10.6%) than females (3.5%), in single patients (10.6%) compared to married ones (2.4%) and in those with lower level of education (17.1%) compared to those with junior high school education or above (2.5%).

3.4. Neoplasms

The MEDLINE search on *Neoplasms* yielded 359 hits, of which 25 reports were ordered. Of these, 12 reports were included as epidemiological studies on the association between schizophrenia and cancer. A further 27 reports were identified by cross-referencing.

Research on the association between schizophrenia and cancer has a long history, and so has the hypothesis of a decreased cancer risk in schizophrenia. An early review by du Pan and Muller (1977) quoted 28 studies, the first one published as early as 1909 (Commission of Lunacy for England and Wales 1909, cited by Scheflen 1951). The results conflicted with several studies showing a decreased risk of cancer in schizophrenia, others showing no difference in risk and yet others even showing an increased risk. These early studies were, however, usually based on small numbers, while Baldwin (1979) estimated in a frequently quoted paper that 100 000 person–years are necessary to assess the comorbidity of schizophrenia and cancer. Also, the early studies often used inappropriate statistical techniques. For example, proportional mortality rates were calculated in many of them, i.e. the ratio of cancer deaths to all deaths. This technique underestimates the true cancer risk, as it is the case in schizophrenia that many patients die for other reasons, e.g. suicide or other diseases. In addition, mortality studies are problematic, because cancer mortality is a combination of the susceptibility to develop cancer and the ability to survive the disease. A good survey of the statistical problems of these early studies has been presented by Fox and Howell (1974).

Therefore, incidence studies rather than mortality studies were requested (du Pan and Muller 1977), and a number of such trials have been conducted since the early 1970s. Since the current scientific debate focuses entirely on these recent incidence studies rather than on the old publications, their results will be summarized in the following passages. All were based on the entire population of the respective country (i.e. they were population based). Further details are presented in Table 3.2.

The debate on the early studies of the association between cancer and schizophrenia inspired the World Health Organization to sponsor large studies in five centres – Aarhus (Denmark), Honolulu (Hawaii), Oxford (UK), Rochester (USA) and Nagasaki (Japan). While we are not aware of the final reports of the studies in Oxford and Rochester, the results of the other three centres have been summarized in a publication (Gulbinat *et al.* 1992). The results of the Danish study have also been described elsewhere in more detail (Mortensen 1989). Although all three studies were linking studies, the specific methods and especially the available case registers differed, which may be one explanation why the results in the three centres were not uniform. While the largest cohort in Denmark showed a decreased cancer incidence in men with schizophrenia, the women of Japanese origin in the Honolulu study had an

Table 3.2. Incidence studies on the association between schizophrenia and cancer

Study	Country	Period of observation	Method	Number patients with schizophrenia (S), Control group (C)	Cancer incidence	Data source on Schizophrenia and Cancer	Main results
Nakane and Ohta 1986	Japan (Nagasaki)	1960–78	Linkage of Nagasaki register of schizophrenia and Nagasaki register of malignant neoplasms	S: 3107 (1717 men, 1388 women)[a], C: general population of Nagasaki	Rel. R – all: 1.5 (n.s.), men: 1.4 (n.s.), women: 1.7 (n.s.)	Nagasaki Medical Association Tumor Statistical Committee, all psychiatric institutions and Nagasaki Mental Health Center	Higher risk of cancer, but not statistically significant
Mortensen 1989	Denmark	1957–84	Incidence of cancer in a cohort of schizophrenic inpatients in one Danish psychiatric hospital. The incidence of cancer (IRR) in the study population was calculated by using the person–years method	S: 6152 (2956 men, 3196 women), C: general population of Denmark	IRR – all: 0.90 (s), men: 0.76 (s.), women: 1.06 (n.s.)	Danish Psychiatric Central Register, Danish Cancer Register	The overall incidence rate of cancer was significantly reduced in all patients and in men while women did not differ from the general population. Surprisingly, a substantial part of the risk reduction was due to lung cancer. Results on specific cancer sites were mixed

Study	Country	Period	Aim	Sample	Results	Register	Conclusions
Gulbinat et al. 1992	USA (Honolulu)	1962–80		S: 6977 (4198 men, 2779 women), C: general population of Honolulu	RR – Honolulu Caucasian – men: 1.00 (n.s), women: 0.62 (n.s.); Honolulu Japanese – men: 1.21 (n.s.), women: 1.73 (n.s.)	Hawaii State Psychiatric Register	Increased cancer risk in women of Japanese origin, but not statistically significant. No difference in Japanese males or Caucasians of either sex
Mortensen 1994	Denmark	1970–87	Incidence of cancer in all first admitted patients in Denmark with a diagnosis of schizophrenia	S: 9156, C: general population of Denmark	SIR – all: 0.79 (s.), men: 0.58 (s.), women: 0.86 (n.s.)	Danish Central Psychiatric Register, Danish Cancer Register, Danish Central Person Registry	Reduced overall incidence of cancer, particularly in men. No significant reduction in women. No type of cancer occurred with a significantly increased rate. Smoking adjusted SIR (SIR = 0.60, no CI indicated) showed even more marked the reduced cancer incidence in schizophrenic patients

Table 3.2. (*cont.*)

Study	Country	Period of observation	Method	Number patients with schizophrenia (S), Control group (C)	Cancer incidence	Data source on Schizophrenia and Cancer	Main results
Lawrence et al. 2000	Australia	1982–95	Investigation of the association between mental illness and cancer incidence, mortality and case fatality. Calculation of the RateR	Patients with mental illness: 172 932 (men 78 228, women 94 704), S: 9997 (males 5656, females 4341), C: general population of Western Australia	RateR – men: 0.83 (s.), women: 1.13 (n.s.)	Western Australia Health Services Research Linked Database, Western Australia Cancer Register	Lower cancer incidence rates in men with schizophrenia, no effect in women. However, significantly higher cancer mortality and case fatality in psychiatric patients (numbers for schizophrenia patients not indicated separately)
Lichtermann et al. 2001	Finland	1971–96	Cancer incidence in patients with schizophrenia born between 1940 and 1969 and their non-psychotic siblings and parents. Calculation of the SIR	S: 26 996 (men 15 578, women 11 418), parents: 39 131, siblings: 52 976, C: general population of Finland	SIR – all: 1.17 (s.), men: 1.25 (s.), women: 1.12 (s.)	National Hospital Discharge and Disability Pension Register of Finland, Finnish Cancer Registry, Central Population Register of Finland	Increased overall cancer risk in schizophrenic patients. Half of the excess cases: lung cancer (SIR = 2.17, s.). However, reduced risk in siblings (SIR = 0.89, s.) and parents (SIR = 0.91, s.)

Author	Country	Period	Aim	Sample	Results	Source	Conclusion
Cohen et al. 2002	USA		Risk of cancer among schizophrenic persons, controlling for known risk and demographic factors (age, race, gender, marital status, education, net worth, smoking and hospitalization in the year before death). Calculation of OR	S: 130, C: 18 603	OR: 0.62 (s.)	1986 National Mortality Followback Survey in the USA, hospital records, death certificates in the USA, interview protocols	Reduced risk of cancer. Increased association (OR: 0.59, s.) after controlling for factors including age, socioeconomic status and smoking
Dalton et al. 2004	Denmark	1969–97	Risk of cancer in parents of patients with schizophrenia	Parents of schizophrenics: 19 856, C: 1 999 072 parents of children without schizophrenia	RR – Fathers of S: 1.01 (n.s.), mothers of S: 1.00 (n.s.)	Danish Psychiatric Central Register, Danish Cancer Registry, Danish Central Population Registry	Overall, no difference in risk of cancer in parents of schizophrenic patients
Grinshpoon et al. 2005	Israel	1962–2001	Association of schizophrenia and cancer in	S: 33 372, C: general population of Israel	SIR – men: 0.86 (s.), women: 0.91 (s.)	Psychiatric Case Register of Israel, Israeli	Reduced risk for all cancer sites for the combined ethnic

Table 3.2. (*cont.*)

Study	Country	Period of observation	Method	Number patients with schizophrenia (S), Control group (C)	Cancer incidence	Data source on Schizophrenia and Cancer	Main results
			Jewish Israelis (age: 15–45 years), comparison of three population groups with respect to their place of origin: Israel-born, Europe–America, Africa–Asia			Cancer Register	groups of patients with schizophrenia. However, higher risk of cancer in persons with schizophrenia than in the general population in specific sites: lung in men, and the corpus uteri and breast in women
Barak *et al.* 2005	Israel	1993–2003	Incidence of cancer in patients with schizophrenia compared with the expected incidence in an age- and gender-matched general population sample	S: 3226, C: General Jewish population of Israel	SIR: 0.58 (s.)	Computerized health registry of Abarbanel Mental Health Center, Israeli National Cancer Registry	Significantly reduced risk for all cancers in patients with schizophrenia. Significantly reduced risk for breast cancer (SIR = 0.61, s.) and skin cancer (SIR = 0.40, s.)

| Dalton et al. 2005 | Denmark | 1960–93 | Risk of cancer in patients with schizophrenia | S: 22 766, C: general population of Denmark | SIR – all: 0.98 (n.s.), men: 0.85 (s.), women: 1.03 (n.s.) | Danish Psychiatric Central Register, Danish Central Population Register | No difference in the overall risk for cancer. Decreased risk for all cancers in men. In women, no significantly decreased risk for any cancer, but increased risk for breast cancer (SIR = 2.59, s.). |
| Goldacre et al. 2005 | UK | 1963–99 | Cancer rates in people with schizophrenia compared with a non-psychiatric reference group | S: 9649, C: nearly 600 000 patients with various medical and surgical conditions | Adjusted[b] RR: 0.99 (n.s.) | Oxford Record Linkage Study | The overall risk ratio for all cancer was not different to the general population |

CI, confidence interval; IRR, incidence rate ratio; n.s., not statistically significant; OR, odds ratio; RateR, rate ratio; RR, relative risk; SIR, standardized incidence rate (observed/expected number of cases standardized for age and sex); s., statistically significant. RR, SIR, IRR < 1 = decreased incidence; RR, SIR, IRR > 1 = increased incidence.

[a] In two patients gender was not indicated.
[b] Adjusted for gender, age in 5-year bands and time period in single calendar years.

increased risk, and the results from Nagasaki lay somewhere in between. In terms of specific cancer sites, the most surprising finding was the decreased risk of lung cancer in the Danish study, because it is nowadays well established that high numbers of smokers can be found among people with schizophrenia (de Leon and Diaz 2005, Masterson and O'Shea 1984). The main – anecdotal – explanation for this striking finding was that smoking was prohibited in Danish hospitals at that time and that these often long-time hospitalized patients were so poor that they could not afford cigarettes. Other suggestions that had been proposed by investigators to explain hypotheses on decreased/increased cancer risk in schizophrenia are summarized in Table 3.3. One of them, the notion that neuroleptics protect against cancer, found some support in a further analysis of the Danish cohort (Mortensen 1987).

The potential confounding factor of smoking prohibition led Mortensen's group to conduct another population-based linkage study analysing a more recent cohort of 9156 patients who were first admitted to hospital when smoking was generally allowed in Danish hospitals (Mortensen 1994). This study confirmed the decreased risk of cancer in patients with schizophrenia. Please note that the samples of the studies by the Danish group around Mortensen partly overlapped and can therefore not be strictly considered to be independent. When smoking was controlled for, the decrease was even more pronounced. Since reduced smoking could thus not explain the findings, Mortensen speculated in line with previous researchers that an antitumour activity of phenothiazines that seems to be well documented in animal experiments (Jones 1985) may explain the decreased risk. The main methodological problem discussed by the authors was that the relatively young age of the patients included led to a low baseline risk for cancer.

The Australian study by Lawrence *et al.* (2000) again found a decreased risk of cancer in men with schizophrenia, while in women there was a trend toward an increased risk. The authors also discuss their findings as an expression of the antitumour effects of antipsychotics which may reduce the cancer risk in men, while an increase of female hormones, e.g. prolactin, may counter this protection in women. The latter assumption was, however, not confirmed by a further Danish linkage study on breast cancer in which the overall risk did not differ from non-schizophrenic women and which showed an effect of parity (Dalton *et al.* 2003). The authors describe this finding as an important argument that antipsychotic drugs do not increase the risk of breast cancer from an epidemiological point of view although they did not control for the use of medication in their study. A crucial additional finding of the Australian study was that psychiatric patients had higher case fatality rate ratios for cancer. This means that once a psychiatric patient develops a cancer, his chances of being cured are lower than those of 'normal' people, highlighting the problem that psychiatric patients probably have worse access to services.

Table 3.3. Hypotheses to explain the association between cancer and schizophrenia

Environmental	Pharmacological	Biochemical	Psychosomatic
	Explanation		
Better or worse diet in hospital[j, k, l]	Antitumor activity of phenothiazines[d, h, i, l]	Inborn deficiency of schizophrenics to utilize methionine as donor of labile methyl groups[c, l]	Old theory that is currently not followed by most experts in the field[c, l]
Reduced exposure to occupational carcinogens[a]	Prolactin increase induced by antipsychotics possibly associated with breast cancer[h]		
Better access to medical care when hospitalized versus less access to services in general[g, l]		Other unknown genetic factor that leads to schizophrenia on the one hand but protects from cancer on the other[f, h]	
Reduced sexual activity (important in breast and cancer of the cervix)[a, b, c, l]			
Less exposure to sun[e, h, j]			

[a] Mortensen 1989.
[b] Dupont *et al.* 1986.
[c] du Pan and Muller 1977.
[d] Mortensen 1992.
[e] Mortensen 1994.
[f] Lichtermann *et al.* 2001.
[g] Dalton *et al.* 2003.
[h] Grinshpoon *et al.* 2005.
[i] Dalton *et al.* 2005.
[j] Goldacre *et al.* 2005.
[k] Barak *et al.* 2005.
[l] Cohen *et al.* 2002.

Further support for a lower incidence of cancer in schizophrenia was provided by an American study that was a combined incidence/mortality study (Cohen *et al.* 2002). It was population based and controlled for factors such as age, but analysed only a random sample of 1% of all deaths that occurred in the United States in 1986, so that the number of people with schizophrenia was low ($n = 130$).

Grinshpoon *et al.* (2005) found a significantly lower cancer risk in both men and women with schizophrenia. However, in contrast to some of the previous studies, especially those from Denmark, the rate of lung cancer was significantly increased in men.

Dalton *et al.* (2005 investigated the cancer risk of 22 766 adults admitted for schizophrenia in Denmark and compared the result with national incidence rates. Their study supported the hypothesis of a decreased risk for cancer among male patients with schizophrenia, including tobacco-related cancers. Significantly decreased risks were found for prostate cancer and cancer of the rectum in male patients. A significantly increased risk for breast cancer found for female patients with schizophrenia should be interpreted with caution, given the high proportion of nulliparous women with schizophrenia in Denmark.

Goldacre *et al.* (2005) linked hospital and deaths records from the Oxford Record Linkage Study (Goldacre *et al.* 2000) to compare cancer rates in people with schizophrenia with a general population reference cohort. The cancer rates did not differ from the rates in the general population.

Finally, the most recent contribution was a population-based incidence study from Israel by Barak *et al.* (2005). The results demonstrated a significantly reduced risk of cancer (all tumour sites together) in patients with schizophrenia.

Thus, although these studies differed in the exact numbers presented, in risks for specific cancer sites (where the number of people included were often too low to allow robust findings) and in their interpretation, most of them supported a reduced risk of cancer in general. These studies were seriously challenged by a Finnish population-based incidence study, which was the largest study in terms of person–years of risk and showed an increased risk of cancer in both men and women; and half of the excess cases were attributable to lung cancer (in contrast to the Danish studies where even lung cancer was reduced). The authors speculated that these findings could be in part due to the fact that smoking was never prohibited in Finnish hospitals, although this argument does not appear to be compelling because the second Danish study had ruled out this confounder (Mortensen 1994). Even more peculiar was the finding that although the cancer risk of people with schizophrenia was increased, the risk of their siblings and parents was decreased. The latter finding was in favour of a theory of a genetic factor protecting from schizophrenia which may be overridden by risk increasing factors such as smoking and alcohol abuse common in these patients. But then Dalton *et al.* (2004) challenged the latter finding by comparing parents of people with schizophrenia with *parents* among the normal population rather than comparing them with the normal population *in general* where no reduction of risk was found.

In summary, after 100 years of research this epidemiological question remains unsolved. Although it could be stated that the majority of the most recent and methodologically best studies found a decreased cancer incidence in people with schizophrenia, counting of studies is inappropriate. The largest study in size (Lichtermann *et al.* 2001) found an increased risk and in terms of specific cancer sites the single studies showed in part contradictory results. It appears that there are also no obvious methodological reasons explaining the differences. Although with few exceptions the studies discussed were population based and were studies which linked psychiatric and cancer registers, the exact methods used and the types of the underlying registers differed. All authors discuss general potential biases of epidemiological studies, namely a different (lower) detection of cancers in people with schizophrenia for example due to less frequent autopsies compared to the general population and the completeness of the registers used. All authors provide good reasons why these factors did not bias their results. A joint discussion paper on the different groups and their results and methods might still be useful. In addition Grinshpoon *et al.* (2005) called for an international epidemiological study with a uniform methodology that would take ethnic differences into account. But from the perspective of the increased general mortality of people with schizophrenia (Brown *et al.* 1999) the most important finding may be the one from the Australian study, namely that although the cancer incidence was reduced, cancer mortality was increased in schizophrenia. This suggests that even if people with schizophrenia were protected by some factor from contracting cancer, their likelihood of being cured of cancer is reduced. Since this is probably explained by the lower access of the mentally ill to medical services (Coghlan *et al.* 2001, Lawrence *et al.* 2000), more research in this direction is warranted.

3.5. Musculoskeletal diseases

The MEDLINE search on *Musculoskeletal Diseases* yielded 316 hits. From these 26 reports were ordered, of which five were included; 20 reports were added by cross-referencing.

A number of studies examined antipsychotic-induced hyperprolactinaemia. Since hyperprolactinaemia is only a laboratory value, but not a comorbid disease in the proper sense, these studies will not be reviewed here. This review focuses on comorbid diseases rather than on side-effects of medication, although the separation is not always clear.

The rest of the studies were on osteoporosis. Given the importance of this comorbidity we made a supplemental MEDLINE search which yielded another 40 hits, of which four were included. Further studies were added by cross-referencing.

Some physiological facts may be useful for the psychiatric reader. Prolactin is secreted by the anterior pituitary gland in a pulsatile manner. Daytime levels and peak amplitudes vary considerably between individuals, and in women levels are higher at the middle of and during the second half of the menstrual cycle. Transient and mild increases of prolactin secretion occur in response to meals, stress and sexual activity. The upper limit of unstimulated prolactin levels in men and women varies between laboratories, ranging between 350 and 550 mU/l (Wieck and Haddad 2003). Prolactin has effects on lactation, gonadal function, reproductive behaviour, and also possibly angiogenesis, osmoregulation and regulation of the immune system (Meaney and O'Keane 2002).

Bone strength is determined by bone mineral density (BMD) which accounts for about 70% of bone strength and bone quality. This index is a proxy measure for bone strength (National Institutes of Health 2004) and is expressed in grams of mineral per area or volume. An individual's BMD is determined by peak bone mass achieved during the first two decades of life and subsequent amount of bone loss (Naidoo *et al.* 2003). Some 80% of the variance of peak bone mass is genetically determined. The remaining variance is caused by the interaction of hormones, nutrition, lifestyle and environmental factors (Cohen and Roe 2000).

3.5.1. Osteoporosis

Osteoporosis is defined as a BMD of more than 2.5 standard deviations below the mean value for peak bone mass in young adults when measured by dual-energy X-ray absorptiometry (DEXA) (Council of the National Osteoporosis Foundation 1996). The most common primary form of bone loss is post-menopausal and age-related osteoporosis. The most common secondary form of bone loss is drug-induced osteoporosis (Hummer *et al.* 2005). Prolactin-increasing antipsychotics are regularly mentioned as a risk factor for osteoporosis. While many conventional antipsychotic drugs substantially increase prolactin levels, some atypical antipsychotics do not or increase them only transiently (aripiprazole, clozapine, quetiapine, olanzapine, ziprasidone, zotepine). Amisulpride and risperidone are two exceptions here, because they increase prolactin levels even more than haloperidol. Antipsychotic-induced elevations of prolactin levels are caused by blockage of dopamine 2 (D2) receptors in the hypothalamic–pituitary axis, which may lead to hypogonadism in both men and women. In women, a chronic prolactin elevation induces inhibition of the hypothalamic secretion of luteinizing-hormone-releasing hormone. This, in turn, lowers luteinizing hormone (LH) and follicle-stimulating hormone (FSH) levels, which regulate gonadal steroid production and release (Halbreich *et al.* 2003). The resulting oestrogen deficiency may reduce bone density in women (Klibanski *et al.* 1980). In men, hypogonadism has also been shown to be a major risk factor for osteoporosis (Stanley *et al.* 1991). Testosterone deficiency has been shown to be associated with profound osteopenia. Some other androgens might be involved in this process, but osteoporosis is less studied in men than in women (Halbreich and Palter 1996). Halbreich and Palter (1996) suggested that the decrease in BMD in untreated as well as medicated patients with schizophrenia might be attributed to multiple accumulated disease- and medication-related processes: negative symptoms, sedentary lifestyle and lack of exercise, hyperprolactinaemia, hypogonadism, increased interleukin activity, polydipsia and impaired fluid and electrolyte balance, alcohol and drug abuse and heavy smoking, dietary and vitamin deficiencies, decreased exposure to sunshine.

In the following the identified studies on the prevalence of loss of bone mineral density in patients with schizophrenia are summarized.

Baastrup *et al.* (1980) measured bone mineral content (BMC) in both forearms in 50 schizophrenic patients receiving antipsychotic drugs compared with 712 age- and sex-matched control subjects. The mean BMC value was 86% of normal ($p < 0.001$), and the decrease was independent of the type of antipsychotic treatment. In contrast, biochemical variables (serum calcium, magnesium, phosphate and alkaline phosphatases) were normal. Baastrup and colleagues recommended further studies including measurements of parathyroid hormone and vitamin D metabolism to clarify the pathogenesis underlying the osteopenia in schizophrenics. Furthermore, they suggested longitudinal studies to elucidate whether the disease or the treatment are the cause of the bone loss.

Ataya *et al.* (1988) evaluated bone density and reproductive hormones in ten women with antipsychotic-induced hyperprolactinaemia. Three were amenorrhoeic, seven had oligomenorrhoea. Nine patients had galactorrhoea. Bone mineral density was at about the 90th percentile when compared with that in age-, gender-, ethnicity- and weight-matched controls, and it correlated with the vaginal maturation score, a measure of oestrogen exposure.

Delva *et al.* (1989) studied ten male chronic schizophrenic patients with polydipsia and ten non-polydipsic schizophrenic controls matched for gender, diagnosis, duration of illness, age and race to estimate bone density of the lumbar spine and radius and to measure urinary electrolyte excretion. Bone density was abnormally low in the polydipsic group, which also had a markedly increased incidence of fractures (50%). Increased urinary sodium and calcium excretion occurred in the polydipsic group. Delva and colleagues suggested that urinary calcium excretion appears to play a major part in the aetiology of osteopenia. They recommended studies on calcium balance, measurement of parathyroid hormone levels, assessment of vitamin D and its metabolites, and urinary hydroxyproline excretion.

Halbreich *et al.* (1995) measured BMD in 33 female and 35 male medicated psychiatric patients. All patients, but surprisingly especially male patients, had a highly significant decrease in BMD when compared with age- and sex-matched normal data. Halbreich and colleagues detected compression fractures in eight out of 35 psychiatric patients. They found that men had a significant increase in prolactin and sex-hormone-binding globulin and a decrease in LH and free testosterone index. Although the prolactin levels did not correlate with the BMD, Halbreich *et al.* (1995) suggested that reduced BMD may be related to low levels of gonadal hormones, especially in male patients.

Keely *et al.* (1997) studied the prevalence and severity of bone mineral loss and its relationship to sex hormone levels in 16 men aged between 19 to 62 years on long-term antipsychotic treatment. Keeley and colleagues found lower BMD than in age-matched controls. They found a statistically significant increase in prolactin and sex-hormone-binding globulin and a decrease in LH and free testosterone index in the treated versus the control subjects. Prolactin levels did not correlate with BMD.

Bergemann *et al.* (2001) investigated 69 premenopausal, regularly menstruating schizophrenic women aged between 18 and 45 years and 68 age- and sex-matched controls and found a high bone turnover but normal spine and hip BMD.

Zhang-Wong and Seeman (2002) published preliminary results of a study in progress, a survey of women under 45 with schizophrenia in long-term treatment with antipsychotic medication on the prevalence of amenorrhoea, hyperprolactinaemia and risk for osteoporosis. Up to the present, the only finding was that there were no irregular menstrual periods in 27 antipsychotic-treated women. The aim of the study is to recruit 200 premenopausal women in all.

Bilici *et al.* (2002) examined 75 patients with schizophrenia and compared them with 20 healthy controls. They found that patients with antipsychotic medication had lower BMD compared to healthy controls. There was a negative association between the duration of antipsychotic treatment, duration of the illness and BMD. They suggested that some atypical antipsychotics may be safer than the classical antipsychotics in terms of reduced BMD.

Abraham *et al.* (2003) investigated the effect of elevated serum prolactin levels on BMD and bone metabolism in 14 female patients with schizophrenia. They reported an inverse relationship between prolactin levels and bone mass. They measured bone metabolism for a period of 12 months. Higher rates of bone formation and resorption were found in patients with high prolactin levels, but the results did not show an association between elevated prolactin and accelerated BMD loss. Possibly longer time periods are necessary before the metabolic processes become uncoupled and lead to BMD loss.

Meaney *et al.* (2004) studied 55 patients with prolactin-raising antipsychotic medication for more than 10 years. They found age-related reduced BMD in 57% of the male and 32% of the female patients. Higher doses of medication were associated with increased rates of both hyperprolactinaemia and BMD loss. Bone loss was correlated with medication dose and for men, bone loss was inversely correlated with testosterone values.

Liu-Seifert *et al.* (2004) found low bone density in a chronic psychiatric population ($n = 402$) treated with prolactin-elevating antipsychotics. Low bone density was found in 23.2% of the females and in 31.0% of the males. Age and hyperprolactinaemia appear to be risk factors for both men and women.

A cross-sectional study by Hummer *et al.* (2005) examined the BMD of 75 patients with schizophrenia under antipsychotic medication between the ages of 19 and 50. The BMD was significantly lower in the lumbar region in men but not in women with schizophrenia. In male patients, BMD showed a negative correlation with negative symptoms and a positive correlation with

25-hydroxy-vitamin D_3 levels and body mass index (BMI). In female patients, there was a positive correlation between BMI and BMD. Exposure to prolactin-increasing antipsychotics was not related to BMD. They quoted Hafner *et al.* (1994) who explained the sex differences of BMD in schizophrenic patients by the fact that the onset of the disorder is about 5 years earlier in male than in female patients, so that male patients are exposed for a longer time to illness-related factors that may contribute to loss of BMD (Hummer *et al.* (2005)).

Kishimoto *et al.* (2005) measured BMD in 133 female inpatients aged between 20 and 81 years with schizophrenia and compared them with 79 healthy controls. In all age groups except for the 3–4-year-olds and the 4–9-year-olds, the patient population showed a significant reduction in BMD compared with healthy controls.

O'Keane and Meaney (2005) examined premenopausal women with a diagnosis of schizophrenia who exclusively received either prolactin-raising antipsychotic medication ($n = 26$) or prolactin-sparing antipsychotic medica-tion/olanzapine ($n = 12$). There were significantly higher rates of low BMD values in the prolactin-raising group (65%) compared with the olanzapine group (17%).

In summary, the studies identified consistently showed that the loss of BMD is prevalent in schizophrenia. Although this finding is robust, the samples in the single studies were usually small. Population-based studies do not exist, but would be warranted to assess the global impact of the phenomenon. It also appears that despite the increased risk, psychiatrists do not take sufficient care in treating their patients. Bishop *et al.* (2004) investigated whether osteoporo-sis screening, prevention management and/or drug therapy were consistently provided both to women with schizophrenia and to women without schizophre-nia. They found that women with schizophrenia ($n = 46$) aged 45 and older did not receive the same level of osteoporosis care as that of age-matched controls ($n = 46$).

Zhang-Wong and Seeman (2002) presented a rather comprehensive list of recommendations for osteoporosis prevention:

Primary prevention of osteoporosis: smoking cessation, regular weight bearing activity, adequate vitamin D and calcium intake, adequate protein diet (soy, tofu products and sweet potatoes), fruits and vegetables, moderate salt and caffeine intake (Atkinson and Ward 2001).

Secondary prevention of osteoporosis: estrogen replacement therapy (if no coun-terindication), consider alendronate, raloxifene, intranasal calcitonin.

Tertiary prevention of osteoporosis: advise footwear, canes, walkers, prevent house-hold falls by houseproofing, ensure safety of fall and winter walking on driveways and sidewalks.

Furthermore, it has been suggested that patients with traditional antipsy-chotic or risperidone-treatment should be monitored closely to prevent side-effects on bone (Dickson and Glazer 1999).

3.6.   Digestive system diseases

The MEDLINE search on *Digestive System Diseases* yielded 359 hits. From these 34 reports were ordered, of which 15 were included; 19 were added by cross-referencing.

3.6.1.   Coeliac disease

Interest in the role of gluten in the pathogenesis of schizophrenia has been stimulated by reports of beneficial effects of cereal-free, milk-free diets in the treatment of schizophrenic patients (Dohan and Grasberger 1973, Dohan *et al*. 1969, Singh and Kay 1976). Some later studies supported an aetiological association between coeliac disease and schizophrenia while others disputed it. Although these were studies on the aetiology of schizophrenia rather than comorbidity studies, this scientifically interesting issue will be reviewed briefly below.

Stimulated by Dohan's hypothesis, Stevens *et al*. (1977) screened 380 schizophrenic inpatients for the presence of reticulin antibodies and compared them with 153 symptomatic patients and 64 untreated coeliac patients. The incidence of reticulin antibodies was similar in schizophrenic patients and controls so that the hypothesis of a positive genetic relationship between schizophrenia and coeliac disease was rejected. Further negative studies were those by McGuffin *et al*. (1981) and Lambert *et al*. (1989).

McGuffin *et al*. (1981) found no differences between the distribution of antibody titres of coeliac disease in patients with schizophrenia ($n = 31$), patients with affective disorders ($n = 29$) and normal controls ($n = 30$).

Lambert *et al*. (1989) investigated small-intestine permeability in 24 patients with schizophrenia and compared it to patients with coeliac disease and normal controls. They found no differences between the groups.

Some support for a link between schizophrenia and coeliac disease was provided by Perisic *et al*. (1990). They analysed the family records of 554 coeliac children. There were three children with schizophrenic parents. Two of the children had autism-like symptoms, the third child was negativistic and irritable. After starting a gluten-free diet, their mental status improved dramatically, suggesting a link between the two disorders. Perisic and colleagues discussed the idea that children of schizophrenic patients may have an increased risk for coeliac disease, but the design of the study and the low number of patients with some schizophrenia-like symptoms can not be considered to be a proof.

Eaton *et al*. (2004) concluded from a population-based case control study that coeliac disease might be a risk factor for schizophrenia. Among 7997 people with schizophrenia, four patients, and eight parents of patients, had coeliac disease before the patient entered a psychiatric facility. In a comment on this article

Campbell and Foley (2004) pointed out that the relationship was overestimated, because the patients' parents' coeliac status was included in the data, as well. Furthermore, the prevalence of coeliac disease in the Danish population in the years 1989–98 was underestimated. Due to better diagnostic tests nowadays available, the prevalence of coeliac disease in the Danish population should be higher than was estimated.

In summary there is currently no firm proof of an association between schizophrenia and coeliac disease. If there were, this could have important consequences, because gluten-free diets would be a therapeutic possibility for some patients. There is continuing interest in this association (Martinez-Bermejo and Polanco 2002) and even recent case reports demonstrate that there are cases with coeliac disease whose psychiatric symptoms disappear after commencing a gluten-free diet (De Santis *et al.* 1997). Treatment is based on the early recognition of the disorder, which is difficult to infer when there are no gastrointestinal symptoms present.

3.6.2. Acute appendicitis

In a population-based case-control study in Denmark Ewald *et al.* (2001) compared the prevalence of acute appendicitis in schizophrenia with that in normal control subjects and in manic-depressive psychosis. Compared to normal controls, patients with schizophrenia had a reduced relative risk of acute appendicitis of 0.49 before and of 0.59 after first psychiatric admission. Multiple interpretations of the negative association were discussed (genetic factors, lifestyle, hospitalization, psychiatric treatment, decreased pain sensitivity and others).

The Oxford Record Linkage Study published by Baldwin (1979) also found a significantly decreased relative risk (0.14) of appendicitis in women with schizophrenia.

Lawrence *et al.* (2001) screened 3368 schizophrenic male patients and 1674 female schizophrenic patients in Western Australia from 1989 to 1998. They found a reduced first-time hospitalization rate ratio for appendicitis of 0.70 (s) in males and 0.85 (n.s.) in females.

Lauerma *et al.* (1998) investigated the inverse relationship: the incidence rate of schizophrenia in a group of patients with appendicitis was 0.47% compared to 0.96% in 5626 patients with rheumatoid arthritis (RA). These findings were unexpected because RA has been shown to be negatively associated with schizophrenia (see section 3.17). They therefore carried out another study on the prevalence of RA and appendicitis in a Northern Finland birth cohort. The frequencies of RA and appendicitis among the patients with schizophrenia ($n = 76$), those with other psychiatric disorders ($n = 438$) and the control group without a psychiatric diagnosis ($n = 10\,503$) were similar. The results of the initial study could therefore not be confirmed, but the low number of schizophrenic patients limited the generalizability of the findings.

Table 3.4. Cancer of the digestive tract in general

Study	Country	Number of schizophrenic patients	Control group	Incidence rate for cancer of the digestive tract in patients with schizophrenia
Mortensen 1989	Denmark	6152: men 2956, women 3196	General population of Denmark	IRR – men: 0.93 (n.s.), women: 1.16 (s.)
Mortensen 1994	Denmark	9156: men 5658, women 3498	General population of Denmark	SIR – men: 0.53 (s.), women: 0.98 (n.s.)

IRR, incidence rate ratio (observed/expected number of cases standardized for age and sex); n.s., not statistically significant; s., statistically significant; SIR, standardized incidence rate. SIR, IRR < 1 = decreased incidence; SIR, IRR > 1 = increased incidence.

Table 3.5. Cancer of the oesophagus

Study	Country	Number of schizophrenic patients	Control group	Incidence rate for oesophagus cancer in patients with schizophrenia
Mortensen 1989	Denmark	6152: men 2956, women 3196	General population of Denmark	IRR – men: 1.18 (n.s.), women: 1.21 (n.s.)
Lichtermann et al. 2001	Finland	26 996	General population of Finland	SIR – 1.10 (n.s.)
Barak et al. 2005	Israel	3226	General Jewish population of Israel	SIR – 1.89 (n.s.)
Dalton et al. 2005	Denmark	22 766: men 13 023, women 9743	General population of Denmark	SIR – men: 2.28 (s.), women: 1.62 (s.)
Goldacre et al. 2005	UK	9649	600 000 hospital patients in the Oxford Health Region	RR – 1.61 (s.)

IRR, incidence rate ratio (observed/expected number of cases standardized for age and sex); n.s., not statistically significant; RR, relative risk; s., statistically significant; SIR, standardized incidence rate. RR, SIR, IRR < 1 = decreased incidence; RR, SIR, IRR > 1 = increased incidence.

In summary, the available evidence suggests lower rates of appendicitis in people with schizophrenia compared to normal controls. But the reasons for the lower rates are unclear and, for example, underreporting due to decreased pain sensitivity can not be ruled out.

Table 3.6. Cancer of the stomach

Study	Country	Number of schizophrenic patients	Control group	Incidence rate for stomach cancer in patients with schizophrenia
Mortensen 1989	Denmark	6152: men 2956, women 3196	General population of Denmark	IRR – men: 1.20 (n.s.), women: 1.26 (n.s.)
Lawrence *et al.* 2000	Australia	172 932 patients with various psychiatric disorders (number of men and women unknown)	General population of Western Australia	RR – men: 0.86 (n.s.), women: 0.80 (n.s.)
Barak *et al.* 2005	Israel	3226	General Jewish population of Israel	SIR – 0.35 (n.s.)
Dalton *et al.* 2005	Denmark	22 766: men 13 023, women 9743	General population of Denmark	SIR – men: 1.13 (n.s.), women: 0.80 (n.s.)
Goldacre *et al.* 2005	UK	9649	600 000 hospital patients in the Oxford Health Region	RR – 0.84 (n.s.)

IRR, incidence rate ratio (observed/expected number of cases standardized for age and sex); n.s., not statistically significant; RR, relative risk; s., statistically significant; SIR, standardized incidence rate. RR, SIR, IRR < 1 = decreased incidence; RR, SIR, IRR > 1 = increased incidence.

3.6.3. Gastric ulcer

The incidence of peptic ulcer in mentally ill patients has been reported in a controversial manner as well. Investigating the hypothesis that schizophrenia is a biochemical disorder, Hinterhuber and Lochenegg (1975) found a 2.69% incidence of gastric ulcers in 668 male schizophrenic patients in contrast to the average rate of 10% in the general population reported in the literature. Hinterhuber and Lochenegg speculated that an altered hypothalamic stress response might explain the low incidence of gastric ulcers in schizophrenic patients.

In contrast to their findings Hussar (1968) surveyed 1275 autopsy protocols of schizophrenic patients. The incidence of healed and active ulcers was 6% which was within the range of reported incidence rates in the general

Table 3.7. Cancer of the colon

Study	Country	Number of schizophrenic patients	Control group	Incidence rate for colon cancer in patients with schizophrenia
Mortensen 1989	Denmark	6152: men 2956, women 3196	General population of Denmark	IRR – men: 0.81 (n.s.), women: 1.07 (n.s.)
Lawrence et al. 2000	Australia	172 932 patients with various psychiatric disorders (number of men and women unknown)	General population of Western Australia	RR – Men: 0.88 (n.s.), Women: 0.97 (n.s.)
Lichtermann et al. 2001	Finland	26 996	General population of Finland	SIR – 0.86 (n.s.)
Barak et al. 2005	Israel	3226	General Jewish population of Israel	SIR – 0.66 (n.s.)
Dalton et al. 2005	Denmark	22 766: men 13 023, women 9743	General population of Denmark	SIR – men: 0.93 (n.s.), women: 0.96 (n.s.)
Goldacre et al. 2005	UK	9649	600 000 hospital patients in the Oxford Health Region	RR – 0.72 (n.s.)

IRR, incidence rate ratio (observed/expected number of cases standardized for age and sex); n.s., not statistically significant; RR, relative risk; s., statistically significant; SIR, standardized cancer incidence rate. RR, SIR, IRR < 1 = decreased incidence; RR, SIR, IRR > 1 = increased incidence.

population. Viskum (1975) investigated the inverse relationship – the incidence of psychoses in patients with ulcers. There was an excess of patients with neuroses and psychopathy among patients with ulcers. This old literature appears to be inconclusive.

3.6.4. Acute intermittent porphyria

Acute intermittent porphyria is a hereditary deficiency of porphyrin metabolism in which the main metabolic effect is caused by a decrease in porphobilinogen deaminase activity. Stimulated by some old studies showing a high prevalence of

Table 3.8. Cancer of the rectum

Study	Country	Number of schizophrenic patients	Control group	Incidence rate for rectum cancer in patients with schizophrenia
Mortensen 1989	Denmark	6152: men 2956, women 3196	General population of Denmark	IRR – men: 0.81 (n.s.), women: 1.07 (n.s.)
Lawrence et al. 2000	Australia	172 932 patients with various psychiatric disorders (number of men and women unknown)	General population of Western Australia	RR – men: 0.88 (n.s.), women: 0.97 (n.s.)
Lichtermann et al. 2001	Finland	26 996	General population of Finland	SIR – 0.35 (s.)
Barak et al. 2005	Israel	3226	General Jewish population of Israel	SIR – 0.19 (n.s.)
Dalton et al. 2005	Denmark	22 766: men 13 023, women 9743	General population of Denmark	SIR – men: 0.62 (s.), women: 1.22 (n.s.)
Goldacre et al. 2005	UK	9649	600 000 hospital patients in the Oxford Health Region	RR – 0.57 (s.)

IRR, incidence rate ratio (observed/expected number of cases standardized for age and sex); n.s., not statistically significant; RR, relative risk; s., statistically significant; SIR, standardized incidence rate. RR, SIR, IRR < 1 = decreased incidence; RR, SIR, IRR > 1 = increased incidence.

acute intermittent porphyria in psychiatric populations (Kaelbling et al. 1961, Tishler et al. 1985), Jara-Prado et al. (2000) evaluated 300 psychiatric patients and 150 control subjects in Mexico. There was no difference between psychiatric patients and controls.

3.6.5. Irritable bowel syndrome

The prevalence of irritable bowel syndrome (IBS), a functional gastrointestinal disorder, has been reported to be 1–2% in the general population, with a slight

Table 3.9. Cancer of the biliary tract

Study	Country	Number of schizophrenic patients	Control group	Incidence rate for cancer of the biliary tract in patients with schizophrenia
Mortensen 1989	Denmark	6152: men 2956, women 3196	General population of Denmark	IRR – men: 1.60 (n.s.), women: 1.32 (n.s.)
Lichtermann et al. 2001	Finland	26 996	General population of Finland	SIR – 2.07 (s.)
Barak et al. 2005	Israel	3226	General Jewish population of Israel	SIR – 1.17 (n.s.)

IRR, incidence rate ratio (observed/expected number of cases standardized for age and sex); n.s., not statistically significant; s., statistically significant; SIR, standardized incidence rate. SIR, IRR < 1 = decreased incidence; SIR, IRR > 1 = increased incidence.

Table 3.10. Cancer of the liver

Study	Country	Number of schizophrenic patients	Control group	Incidence rate for liver cancer in patients with schizophrenia
Mortensen 1989	Denmark	6152: men 2956, women 3196	General population of Denmark	IRR – men: 0.82 (n.s.), women: 1.11 (n.s.)
Lichtermann et al. 2001	Finland	26 996	General population of Finland	SIR – 1.55 (n.s.)
Dalton et al. 2005	Denmark	22 766: men 13 023, women 9743	General population of Denmark	SIR – men : 1.17 (n.s.), women: 0.99 (n.s.)
Goldacre et al. 2005	UK	9649	600 000 hospital patients in the Oxford Health Region	RR – 1.33 (n.s.)

IRR, incidence rate ratio (observed/expected number of cases standardized for age and sex); n.s., not statistically significant; RR, relative risk; SIR, standardized incidence rate. RR, SIR, IRR < 1 = decreased incidence; RR, SIR, IRR > 1 = increased incidence.

predominance in women (Drossman 1994). Patients seeking medical attention for IBS may have a comorbid psychiatric condition, mainly depression, in 7%–0% of the cases. Only a few studies have considered the prevalence of IBS in psychiatric patients.

Table 3.11. Cancer of the pancreas

Study	Country	Number of schizophrenic patients	Control group	Incidence rate for pancreas cancer in patients with schizophrenia
Mortensen 1989	Denmark	6152: men 2956, women 3196	General population of Denmark	IRR – men: 0.64 (n.s.), women: 1.59 (n.s.)
Mortensen 1994	Denmark	9156: men 5658, women 3498	General population of Denmark	SIR – men: 1.22 (n.s.), women: 0.00 (n.s.)
Lawrence et al. 2000	Australia	172 932 patients with various psychiatric disorders (number of men and women unknown)	General population of Western Australia	RR – men: 1.30 (n.s.), women: 1.12 (n.s.)
Lichtermann et al. 2001	Finland	26 996	General population of Finland	SIR – 1.16 (n.s.)
Dalton et al. 2005	Denmark	22 766: men 13 023, women 9743	General population of Denmark	SIR – men : 0.77 (n.s.), women: 0.64 (n.s.)
Goldacre et al. 2005	UK	9649	600 000 hospital patients in the Oxford Health Region	RR – 0.90 (n.s.)

IRR, incidence rate ratio (observed/expected number of cases standardized for age and sex); n.s., not statistically significant; RR, relative risk; SIR, standardized incidence rate. RR, SIR, IRR < 1 = decreased incidence; RR, SIR, IRR > 1 = increased incidence.

Gupta et al. (1997) compared 47 patients with schizophrenia to 40 age-matched controls. Of the patients with schizophrenia 19% met the criteria for IBS in contrast to 2.5% of the control group. The authors pointed out that people with schizophrenia rarely complain about gastrointestinal symptoms until specifically asked. Therefore prior to starting antipsychotic treatment, psychiatrists should inquire about gastrointestinal problems so that side-effects can be differentiated from pre-existing conditions.

3.6.6. Cancers of the digestive system

Tables 3.4 to 3.11 provide a summary of the prevalence of cancers of the digestive tract among schizophrenic patients that were derived from the population-based studies on cancer in section 3.4. The data are very heterogeneous, with most studies showing no statistically significant differences between groups and a few studies showing increased or decreased rates of specific gastrointestinal cancers. This research suffers from limited statistical power, and its results are inconclusive.

3.6.7. Miscellaneous

Finally, the results of a number of small single studies on miscellaneous topics will be briefly summarized below.

Cadalbert *et al.* (1970) reported three case reports of psychiatric patients with functional megacolon.

Kaplan *et al.* (1970) reported a high incidence of schizophrenia among post-gasterectomy patients who continued to complain of abdominal pain in the absence of demonstrable organic pathology. The study was small.

A hypothesis paper by Kroll (2001) speculated on non-hepatocellular liver dysfunction as a predisposing factor in the pathogenesis of schizophrenia. A study on pain insensitivity by Rosenthal *et al.* (1990) was added to the section on diseases of the nervous system (section 3.10), and studies on the association between schizophrenia and hepatitis have been reviewed in the section on *virus diseases* (section 3.2). Finally, some reports that focussed solely on side-effects of clozapine (weight gain, constipation and increase of hepatic enzymes) and chlorpromazine (hepatotoxicity) (Weinreb *et al.* 1978) are beyond the scope of the review and are therefore not summarized here.

Although the association between schizophrenia and a number of disorders of the digestive system has been investigated in epidemiological studies, none of the results can be considered conclusive.

3.7. Stomatognathic diseases

The MEDLINE search on *Stomatognathic Diseases* yielded 141 hits. Ten reports were ordered and nine of them were included.

3.7.1. Oral dyskinesia

Pryce and Edwards (1966) surveyed 121 female schizophrenic patients on the prevalence of abnormal movements in any part of the body associated with phenothiazine treatment. They suggested that oral dyskinesia observed in elderly schizophrenic women may be associated with a high total intake of phenothiazines.

3.7.2. Dental disease

Thomas *et al.* (1996) evaluated the oral health status of 249 chronic schizophrenic patients. They found that inpatients had greater amounts of dental disease than outpatients. The extent of dental disease was directly related to intensity of schizophrenia, the magnitude of negative symptoms associated with schizophrenia, the length of hospitalization and the dose of chloropromazine.

Velasco *et al.* (1997) assessed the dental health status of 565 institutionalized psychiatric patients (62% with a diagnosis of schizophrenia) in Spain. All patients were taking psychotropic medication. The mean number of caries decayed teeth was 7.9, of missing teeth 17.0 and of filled teeth 0.0. The Decayed, Missing and Filled Teeth score (DMFT) increased significantly with age and length of hospitalization. Female and demented patients had significantly higher DMFT scores. The authors concluded that institutionalized patients with mental illness in Spain have extensive untreated dental disease.

Kenkre and Spadigam (2000) evaluated the prevalence of caries, the oral hygiene status and periodontal health and treatment needs in 153 institutionalized psychiatric patients (63% with schizophrenia) in Goa, India. None of the edentulous patients had dentures; 5% had been referred to emergency dental care during their period of institutionalization; 12% were caries-free; 88% were in need of conservative dental treatment; 5.4% reported a healthy periodontium whereas 16.27% required complex periodontal therapy. The authors recommended providing oral health services on a regular basis for this marginalized patient population.

Lewis *et al.* (2001) quantified the oral health status of 326 hospitalized psychiatric patients (23% with a diagnosis of schizophrenia) in South Wales. The mean age of the patients was 71.1 years and 63% were edentulous. The mean DMFT score was 19.1, compared with the DMFT of the general population, the decay level was similar, but the study population had fewer filled teeth and more missing teeth. The authors concluded that the oral hygiene of the study population was poor and that there were treatment needs mainly for scaling and polishing. There were no significant differences between the subgroups of the study population.

Another report, by Friedlander and Marder (2002), was on the importance of special attention to and empathy with schizophrenic patients by dentists. Schizophrenia impairs the patient's ability to plan and perform oral hygiene procedures, and some antipsychotic medications have adverse orofacial effects such as xerostomia. It is recommended that dentists be familiar with the disease schizophrenia so that adequate cooperation between dentist, patient and psychiatrist is possible.

McCreadie *et al.* (2004) examined the dental health of 428 community-dwelling people with schizophrenia and compared the results with those of the UK general population. Significantly more patients were edentate (−9% vs. −0%) and fewer had more than 20 teeth (70% vs. 83%). More patients had last visited the dentist because of trouble with their teeth, fewer had visited for a check-up. Fewer patients cleaned their teeth daily. The authors recommended that community mental health teams should encourage them to attend their community dentist regularly.

Tang *et al.* (2004) examined the oral health status of 91 Chinese psychiatric patients (80.2% with a diagnosis of schizophrenia) in Hong Kong. The mean age was 44.7 years. Malocclusion was found in 79.1% of patients. The mean number of missing teeth was 9.5. Dental caries was found in 75.3% of patients. Older age and length of illness were significantly associated with poor dental health, and the oral health of chronic psychiatric patients was considerably worse than that of the general population.

In summary, various studies around the world have demonstrated a poor dental status of people with schizophrenia.

3.7.3. Temporomandibular disorders

Velasco-Ortega *et al.* (2005) investigated the prevalence of temporomandibular disorders (TMD) in 50 schizophrenic patients from the Psychiatric Unit at the Virgen Macarena Universitary Hospital of Seville compared with 50 control patients from the School of Dentistry of Seville. They found that 32% of schizophrenic patients showed symptoms of TMD, clicking (24%) and self-correcting blocking (8%), compared with 8% (sounds) of control patients. The authors concluded that schizophrenic patients constitute a high risk population for TMD, because they showed a higher prevalence and severity of TMD.

3.8. Respiratory tract diseases

The MEDLINE search on *Respiratory Tract Diseases* yielded 313 hits. 19 reports were ordered and seven of them were included. 11 reports were added by cross-referencing.

3.8.1. Respiratory health: asthma, bronchitis, upper respiratory tract infections, emphysema, pneumonia, chronic obstructive pulmonary disease

Chafetz *et al.* (2005) examined the health conditions of 271 patients with schizophrenia or schizoaffective disorder (SAD) compared with 510 patients with other psychiatric diagnoses from short-term residential treatment facilities in San Francisco. Of the patients with schizophrenia or SAD 10% had asthma vs. 9.8% of the comparison group, and 6.6% had bronchitis or upper respiratory infections (URI) vs. 6.5%. A significantly higher prevalence was found for emphysema or chronic obstructive pulmonary disease (4.1% vs. 1.8%).

Lawrence *et al.* (2001) screened 3368 schizophrenic male patients and 1674 female schizophrenic patients in Western Australia for selected health conditions. They found a first-time hospitalization rate ratio for pneumonia of 1.23 (n.s.) in males and 1.19 (n.s.) in females; the rate ratio for COPD was 1.14 in males and 1.12 (n.s.) in females. The rate ratio for asthma was 0.49 (s.) in males and 0.93 (n.s.) in females.

In Filik *et al.* (2006) the risks of reporting respiratory symptoms, namely breathlessness, phlegm production and wheeze were significantly higher in people with schizophrenia than in a national sample in the UK. Compared with figures reported in the *Health Survey for England 1993* (Bennett *et al.* 1995), lung function was greatly impaired in patients with schizophrenia. Using FEV_1 (forced expiratory volume), the key measure of lung function, 89.6% of the patients had a lung function less than predicted compared with 47% of healthy men and women. Moreover, 41.9% of the patients could be categorized as outside the normal range, exhibiting low lung function, compared with 9% of the healthy population. The results for the FVC (forced vital capacity) were similar (52.1% had low FVC compared with 6% of the healthy population). In summary, the studies support increased rates of respiratory tract problems in schizophrenia. But given the high rates of smoking in schizophrenia, further studies would be welcome to provide a more complete picture of the problem.

3.8.2. Cancers of the respiratory tract

Tables 3.12–3.15 provide a summary of the cancer studies summarized in the section on Neoplasms (section 3.4) that reported on cancers of the respiratory tract. The results are very heterogeneous, showing differences between studies in regard to gender and direction of the effect (increased or decreased risk).

3.9. Otorhinolaryngologic diseases

The MEDLINE search on *Otorhinolaryngologic Diseases* yielded 169 hits. From these, 12 reports were ordered, of which four were included.

3.9.1. Middle ear disease

Mason and Winton (1995) investigated the rates of middle ear disease in patients with schizophrenia compared with rates in non-psychiatric controls. The

Table 3.12. Cancer of the respiratory tract

Study	Country	Number of schizophrenic patients	Control group	Incidence rate for lung cancer in patients with schizophrenia
Mortensen 1989	Denmark	6152: men 2956, women 3196	General population of Denmark	IRR – men: 0.35 (s.), women: 0.53 (s.)
Mortensen 1994	Denmark	9156: men 5658, women 3498	General population of Denmark	SIR – men: 0.60 (n.s.), women: 1.18 (n.s.)

IRR, incidence rate ratio (observed/expected number of cases standardized for age and sex); n.s., not statistically significant; s., statistically significant; SIR, standardized incidence rate. SIR, IRR < 1 = decreased incidence; SIR, IRR > 1 = increased incidence.

relative risk of middle ear disease in schizophrenia was 1.92 (s.). The authors discussed whether middle ear disease may be an aetiological factor in some cases of schizophrenia. The association was even stronger when the middle ear disease pre-dated the onset of schizophrenia and when cases with a genetic loading for schizophrenia were excluded. Mason and Winton (1995) proposed two speculative mechanisms for the association: (1) the overlying temporal lobe may be damaged by a local inflammation within the middle ear and (2) deafness may predispose to the development of psychotic symptoms by the processes of social isolation, sensory deprivation and interference with attention, perception and communication processes (Cooper 1976). However, the study had some methodological problems: no control for social class, lack of operationalized criteria for the diagnosis of schizophrenia and the diagnosis of ear disease, no control for nosocomial factors.

3.9.2. Vestibular response abnormalities

Levy *et al.* (1983) also speculated that vestibular response abnormalities may be aetiological factors for schizophrenia. They reviewed studies made between 1921 and 1980 and concluded that earlier findings overestimated the role of vestibular disease in schizophrenic patients due to experimental artifacts. Nevertheless they support the hypothesis that abnormalities of the vestibular system may be one out of numerous aetiological factors in schizophrenia.

3.9.3. Deafness

Cooper (1976) reviewed the literature for the relationship between deafness and psychiatric disorders. He found that the prevalence of schizophrenia in the prelingually deaf is similar to that found in the normal population, but that the hard-of-hearing are overrepresented among samples of patients

Table 3.13. Lung cancer

Study	Country	Number of schizophrenic patients	Control group	Incidence rate for lung cancer in patients with schizophrenia
Mortensen 1989	Denmark	6152: men 2956, women 3196	General population of Denmark	IRR – men 0.34 (s.), women: 0.29, (s.)
Mortensen 1994	Denmark	9156: men 5658, women 3498	General population of Denmark	SIR – men: 0.62 (n.s.), women: 1.02 (n.s.)
Lichtermann et al. 2001	Finland	269 96	General population of Finland	SIR – 2.17 (s.)
Lawrence et al. 2003	Australia	172 932 patients with various psychiatric disorders (number of men and women unknown)	General population of Western Australia	RR – men: 1.10 (n.s.), women: 1.10 (n.s.)
Barak et al. 2005	Israel	3226	General Jewish population of Israel	SIR – 0.65 (n.s.)
Dalton et al. 2005	Denmark	22 766: men 13 023, women 9649	General population of Denmark	SIR – men: 0.82 (n.s.), women: 1.17 (n.s.)
Goldacre et al. 2005)	UK	9649	600 000 hospital patients in the Oxford Health Region	RR – 1.18 (n.s.)
Grinshpoon et al. 2005	Israel	26 518 (number of men and women not given)	General population of Israel	SIR–men: 1.38 (s.), women: 0.85 (n.s.)

IRR, incidence rate ratio (observed/expected number of cases standardized for age and sex); n.s., not statistically significant; RR, relative risk; s., statistically significant; SIR, standardized incidence rate. RR, SIR, IRR < 1 = decreased incidence; RR, SIR, IRR > 1 = increased incidence.

suffering from paranoid psychosis in later life. Deafness is a social stigma and it is clear that it can influence the personality. He suggested that predisposed individuals with hearing impairment may have misperception of auditory stimuli and may develop inappropriate associations and give unexpected or bizarre answers. Cooper concluded that deafness may have an aetiological significance

Table 3.14. Cancer of the larynx

Study	Country	Number of schizophrenic patients	Control group	Incidence rate for larynx cancer in patients with schizophrenia
Mortensen 1989	Denmark	6152: men 2956, women 3196	General population of Denmark	IRR – men: 0.25 (s.), women: 1.76 (n.s.)
Lichtermann et al. 2001	Finland	26 996	General population of Finland	SIR – 0.94 (n.s.)
Dalton et al. 2005	Denmark	22 766: men 13 023, women 9743	General population of Denmark	SIR – men: 0.56 (n.s.), women: 0.39 (n.s.)
Goldacre et al. 2005	UK	9649	600 000 hospital patients in the Oxford Health Region	RR – 1.09 (n.s.)

IRR, incidence rate ratio (observed/expected number of cases standardized for age and sex); n.s., not statistically significant; RR, relative risk; s., statistically significant; SIR, standardized incidence rate. RR, SIR, IRR < 1 = decreased incidence; RR, SIR, IRR > 1 = increased incidence.

Table 3.15. Cancer of the pharynx

Study	Country	Number of schizophrenic patients	Control group	Incidence rate for pharynx cancer in patients with schizophrenia
Lichtermann et al. 2001	Finland	26 996	General population of Finland	SIR – 2.60 (s.)
Goldacre et al. 2005	UK	9649	600 000 hospital patients in the Oxford Health Region	RR – 0.95 (n.s.)

n.s., not statistically significant; RR, relative risk; s., statistically significant; SIR, standardized cancer incidence rate (observed/expected number of cases standardized for age and sex). RR, SIR < 1 = decreased incidence; RR, SIR > 1 = increased incidence.

for schizophrenia when it occurs at an early age and when it has a long duration and severity.

In a large cohort study (David *et al.* 1995) of 50 000 male Swedish conscripts linked to the Swedish National Register of Psychiatric Care, the schizophrenia rate among patients with severe hearing loss was 1.81 (s). These authors concluded that hearing impairment increases the risk of schizophrenia by 80% and that it may represent a potentially avoidable aetiological factor.

3.10. Diseases of the nervous system

The MEDLINE search on *Diseases of the Nervous System* yielded 15 170 hits. Many of the articles were on the neurological side-effects of antipsychotic drugs rather than neurological comorbidities of schizophrenia in the proper sense (see below). Furthermore, when reviewing this area the MeSH term of schizophrenia with the term *Diseases of the Nervous System* were not simply combined, but rather with the single categories summarized under *Diseases of the Nervous System*. This procedure led to double-counting of many studies. Otherwise, the total number of hits would have been 7500. Nevertheless, only 31 relevant reports were ordered. Five reports were added by cross-referencing. The following subheadings are the respective subcategories under *Diseases of the Nervous System*.

3.10.1. Folate status

Muntjewerff and Blom (2005) reviewed the published case-control studies on folate levels in the population of patients with schizophrenia and found that none of the seven case-control studies included in this review (325 cases and 560 control subjects in all) explicitly reported on all critical factors in the assessment of folate status. In addition, only three studies found lower plasma folate levels more frequently in patients with schizophrenia compared to controls. Further research on this topic is required to clarify the relationship between folate status and schizophrenia.

3.10.2. Autoimmune diseases of the nervous system

Searching for the term *Autoimmune diseases of the nervous system* yielded 122 hits.

Multiple sclerosis

Two reports by Templer and colleagues examined the geographical similarity of multiple sclerosis and schizophrenia rates.

In 1985 Templer *et al.* (1985) found that the ten states in the USA with the highest schizophrenia rates had significantly higher multiple sclerosis rates than the states with the lowest schizophrenia rates.

In 1988, Templer *et al.* (1988) repeated the same study in 17 Italian districts and found a statistically significant correlation between rates of multiple sclerosis and schizophrenia, with a correlation coefficient of 0.81. They suggested common properties and common aetiologies for explaining the similar geographical distributions: both diseases are chronic and are familial disorders that begin in early adult life and run an irregular course. The possibility of a slow virus infection has been suggested for both.

Myasthenia gravis
An early review by Gittleson and Richardson (1973) found that myasthenia gravis and schizophrenia rarely occur in the same patient, and suggested a possible mutual antagonism of the two diseases. These findings were commented on in two case reports, by Dorrell (1973) and Burkitt and Khan (1973), which were interpreted to imply that myasthenia gravis can cause schizophrenic reactions.

Steiner and Abramsky (1989) discussed an autoimmune hypothesis of schizophrenia. An anti-receptor antibody-mediated hypothesis of schizophrenia has not yet been proven; further research into the possible role of the immune system in the pathogenesis of schizophrenia is warranted.

3.10.3. Autonomic nervous system diseases

Searching for the term *Autonomic nervous system diseases* yielded 28 hits. None was relevant.

3.10.4. Central nervous system diseases

Brain diseases
The term *Brain diseases* yielded 4538 hits.

Epilepsy
Epilepsy can clearly be associated with schizophrenia-like symptoms (for review see Sachdev 1998 and Taylor 2003). For example, in a recent Danish population-based study by Qin *et al.* (2005) the relative risk of schizophrenia in people with a history of epilepsy was significantly elevated (relative risk 2.48). But there is only very limited evidence on the inverse direction, i.e. indicating how many people with schizophrenia suffer from epilepsy (Baldwin 1979, Casadebaig 1997). Such studies may be worthwhile, as there may be a genetic link between both diseases (Qin *et al.* 2005).

Hydrocephalus
A comment by Dewan and Bick (1985) discussed the possible aetiological link between normal-pressure hydrocephalus and psychiatric disorders. They quoted

previous studies (Nyback *et al.* 1982, Oxenstierna *et al.* 1984) which showed that some schizophrenic patients have ventricular enlargement or abnormal cerebrospinal fluid circulation.

Central nervous system infections

The term *Central nervous system infections* yielded 147 hits.

A survey by King *et al.* (1985) investigated the antibody titres of eight neurotropic viruses in 450 psychiatric inpatients and 143 controls. They observed low antibody titres for some of the viruses in psychiatric patients, which they explain by an impaired immune response. Other reports (Conejero-Goldberg *et al.* 2003, Lycke *et al.* 1974, Pelissolo 1997, Torrey and Peterson 1973) also attempted to support the hypothesis of a viral genesis of schizophrenia. None of them was able to prove the increased prevalence of any virus, and more research on the role of viruses is warranted.

Encephalomyelitis

The term *Encephalomyelitis* yielded 15 hits. None was relevant.

High-pressure neurological syndrome

The term *High-pressure neurological syndrome* yielded 1 hit, which was not relevant.

Meningitis

The term *Meningitis* yielded 24 hits. None was relevant.

Movement disorders

The term *Movement disorders* yielded 1099 hits. Most of the publications identified were on the well-known extrapyramidal side-effects (EPS) of antipsychotic drugs rather than on neurological comorbidities proper. A complete review of these side-effects (dystonia, akathisia, parkinsonism, dyskinesia and neuroleptic malignant syndrome) would go beyond the scope of this manuscript. Nevertheless, the prevalence of acute EPS has been reported to span a wide range from 2% to 90% (Casey 1993). The risk of developing EPS depends strongly on patients, drugs and time. For example, elderly patients are much more sensitive to EPS than younger patients. Also, the main advantage of the second-generation ('atypical') antipsychotics is a low propensity to induce EPS, at least compared to high-potency conventional antipsychotics (Leucht *et al.* 1999). But so-called low-potency conventional antipsychotics such as chlorpromazine are also known to have a relatively low risk of inducing acute EPS. Furthermore, the occurrence of acute EPS is dose dependent. The most serious long-term extrapyramidal side-effect is tardive dyskinesia. In a review, annual cumulative incidence rates of tardive dyskinesia have been estimated to be 3%–5% in young adults treated with conventional antipsychotics and to reach 2%–5% after 5 years

(Sachdev 2000). The 1-year incidence under treatment with second-generation antipsychotics appears to be lower (Correll *et al.* 2004). Please note that it is also well established that drug-naïve patients with schizophrenia often show motor symptoms (Fenton 2000, Wolff and O'Driscoll 1999). In a review of 14 studies Fenton estimated a prevalence of spontaneous dyskinesia of 4% in first-episode patients, 12% for patients who had been ill several years but were under the age of 30, 25% for those between 30 and 50 years of age and 40% for those aged 60 years or older (Fenton 2000).

Ocular motility disorders
The term *Ocular motility disorders* yielded 68 hits. None was relevant.

Pneumocephalus
The term *Pneumocephalus* yielded no hits.

Spinal cord diseases
The term *Spinal cord diseases* yielded 58 hits. There were no relevant reports.

3.10.5. Chronobiology disorders

The term *Chronobiology disorders* yielded 2 hits. None was relevant.

3.10.6. Cranial nerve diseases

The term *Cranial nerve diseases* yielded 87 hits. None was relevant.

3.10.7. Demyelinating diseases

The term *Demyelinating diseases* yielded 145 hits.

Metachromatic leukodystrophy
One report, by Galbraith *et al.* (1989), was on the prevalence of *metachromatic leukodystrophy* (MLD) in psychiatric patients. Metachromatic leukodystrophy is a rare inherited neurodegenerative disease and is caused by a deficiency of the enzyme sulphatide sulphatase, also known as arylsulphatase A (ASA). The disease may present as a schizophrenic-like psychosis. No case of MLD in schizophrenia was observed.

Shah and Greenberg (1992) measured the activity of ASA in adult psychiatric patients and in normal volunteers using nitrocatechol sulphate (ASA-NCS) and cerebroside sulphate (ASA-CS) as substrates. They found low levels of ASA-CS activity in a significantly large number of adult psychiatric patients with varying psychiatric manifestations. They speculated that psychiatric patients may be asymptomatic heterozygote carriers of the sulphatidase defect and that behavioural and functional disturbances in these patients may at least in part be related to sulphatidase deficiency. The significance of the ASA-NCS abnormality in psychiatric patients is unclear.

Alvarez *et al.* (1995) also found low ASA activity in six out of 23 patients with presumable schizophrenia; five of them had a clinical history of schizophrenic symptoms. They speculated that the schizophrenic symptoms in these patients might be due to the enzyme deficiency. They concluded that patients with suspected schizophrenia should be screened for the enzyme in order to identify cases of MLD.

Amyotrophic lateral sclerosis
Two reports (Howland 1990, Yase *et al.* 1972) were on amyotrophic lateral sclerosis (AML) and found that schizophrenia-like disorders can be observed during the course of AML.

3.10.8. Nervous system malformations

The term *Nervous system malformations* yielded 44 hits. None was considered to be relevant here, but some were added to the sections on female genital diseases and pregnancy complications (section 3.13) or congenital, hereditary and neonatal diseases and abnormalities (section 3.16).

3.10.9. Nervous system neoplasms

The term *Nervous system neoplasms* yielded 123 hits. There were no relevant studies, because there were no studies that especially focussed on nervous-system cancers.

Table 3.16 provides a summary on the prevalence of brain cancer among schizophrenic patients that was derived from the population-based studies on cancer in section 3.4. The results are inconclusive.

3.10.10.   Neurocutaneous syndrome

The term *Neurocutaneous syndrome* yielded 9 hits. None was relevant.

3.10.11.   Neurodegenerative diseases

The term *Neurodegenerative diseases* yielded 962 hits.

Alzheimer's disease
Three reports were on the association of Alzheimer's disease (AD) and schizophrenia.

Table 3.16. Brain cancer

Study	Country	Number of schizophrenic patients	Control group	Incidence rate for brain cancer in patients with schizophrenia
Mortensen 1989	Denmark	6152: men 2956, women 3196	General population of Denmark	IRR – men: 0.69 (n.s.), women: 1.50 (n.s.)
Lawrence et al. 2000	Australia	172 932 patients with various psychiatric disorders (number of men and women unknown)	General population of Western Australia	RR – men: 2.43 (s.), women: 2.15 (s.)
Barak et al. 2005	Israel	3226	General Jewish population of Israel	SIR – 0.20 (n.s.)
Dalton et al. 2005	Denmark	22 766: men 13 023, women 9743	General population of Denmark	SIR – men: 0.74 (n.s.), women: 0.78 (n.s.)
Goldacre et al. 2005	UK	9649	600 000 hospital patients in the Oxford Health Region	Brain (malignant) RR – 0.74 (n.s.) Brain (benign) RR – 1.32 (n.s.)
Grinshpoon et al. 2005	Israel	26 518 (number of men and women not given)	General population of Israel	SIR – men: 0.56 (s.), women: 0.94 (n.s.)

IRR, incidence rate ratio (observed/expected number of cases standardized for age and sex); n.s., not statistically significant; RR, relative risk; s., statistically significant; SIR, standardized incidence rate. RR, SIR, IRR < 1 = decreased incidence; RR, SIR, IRR > 1 = increased incidence.

Prohovnik et al. (1993) reviewed the consecutive neuropathological records of 544 patients with schizophrenia who were chronically hospitalized in New York State mental institutions. The prevalence of neuropathological diagnoses consistent with AD was 28%. This prevalence rate was considerably higher than that estimated for the general population. When evaluated against age at death, AD findings in schizophrenia rose monotonically from under 5% below age 60 to 50% at age 90 and over. The authors speculated that chronic neuroleptic treatment may play a role in the development of AD. The pathophysiological mechanisms of this association remain to be elucidated.

White and Cummings (1996) examined pathophysiological analogies between schizophrenia and AD and observed a dysfunction of the limbic system and disturbances in the dopamine–acetylcholin axis in both schizophrenia and AD.

Murphy *et al.* (1998) made a retrospective chart review of 51 patients over 55 years on the prevalence of AD in patients with schizophrenia. Only one patient met the neuropathological criteria for AD, resulting in a frequency of 2%, a lower prevalence when compared to the rate of 2.4% in non-psychiatric patients over 65 years old. In contrast to previous reports, Murphy and colleagues concluded that the frequency of AD may be equal to or less than that in the general population. Further research on this issue is warranted.

Parkinsonism

Lawrence *et al.* (2001) screened 260 male schizophrenic patients and 255 female schizophrenic patients in Western Australia from 1980 to 1998. They found a first-time hospitalization rate ratio for Parkinson's disease of 6.53 (n.s.) in male and of 7.78 (n.s.) in female patients.

3.10.12. Neurological manifestations

The term *Neurological manifestations* yielded 5020 hits.

Altered pain perception

Most of the relevant studies were on altered pain perception in patients with schizophrenia (Blumensohn *et al.* 2002, Davis *et al.* 1982, Rosenthal *et al.* 1990, Torrey 1979). The description of this phenomenon has a long history and it had already been described by Bleuler in 1911 and by Kraepelin in 1919 (quoted from Dworkin 1994). A number of impressive case reports on changes in pain responsiveness are available. Singh *et al.* (2006) recently reviewed the literature on this topic and, in addition to multiple case reports and experimental studies, presented ten studies with a somewhat more epidemiological approach (Ballenger *et al.* 1979, Delaplaine *et al.* 1978, Goldfarb 1958, Hussar 1965, Lieberman 1955, Marchand Walter 1955, Marchand Walter *et al.* 1959, Torrey 1979, Varsamis and Adamson 1976, Watson *et al.* 1981). The proportion of schizophrenic patients without pain in the different studies varied from 37% (Marchand Walter *et al.* 1959) to 91% (Torrey 1979). They suggested that pain insensitivity is a trait rather than a state marker for schizophrenia.

Although at first glance there seems to be convincing evidence supporting this finding, two reviews came up with somewhat more critical conclusions (Dworkin 1994, Lautenbacher and Krieg 1994). Although these authors also agreed that an extensive and diverse literature supports the hypothesis that many individuals with schizophrenia are less sensitive to pain than normal individuals, they criticized the fact that most of the experimental studies suffered from a number of methodological shortcomings and that some of them showed conflicting findings. Lautenbacher and Krieg (1994) concluded that instead of speaking of hypalgesic changes in schizophrenia, the findings may also be explained by rather general disturbances in somatosensation or perception. Dworkin (1994) concluded that the available research has provided neither a satisfactory characterization nor a satisfactory explanation of pain insensitivity in schizophrenia.

The following five hypotheses for the pain insensitivity of people with schizophrenia have been suggested by Jakubaschk and Boker (1991). They are:
(1) an expression of motorial inability to react
(2) a consequence of a disorder of consciousness
(3) an analgetic effect of neuroleptic drugs
(4) a basic deficit in schizophrenia
(5) a result of a disturbed psychophysiological development.

Watson *et al.* (1981) quoted other possible explanations for this phenomenon, namely:
(1) a lack of appreciation of or responsiveness to pain stimuli (Bleuler 1911, Geschwind 1977, May 1948, Schneider 1959)
(2) a loss of the *meaning* of pain (Geschwind 1977, Marchand Walter 1955)
(3) asymbolia of pain (Geschwind 1977)
(4) abnormalities in brain levels of serotonin, dopamine, prostaglandins and endorphins, which have been described in schizophrenia as well as modulators of normal pain perception (Creese *et al.* 1976, Horrobin *et al.* 1978, Terenius and Wahlstrom 1978).

Nevertheless, whatever the nature of hypalgesia or dysalgesia in schizophrenia may be, this topic is of utmost importance for this review, because it may in part explain the excess morbidity and mortality found in many areas. The call for further studies of pain in schizophrenia by Singh *et al.* (2006), Dworkin (1994) and Lautenbacher and Krieg (1994) is thus warranted.

3.10.13. Neuromuscular diseases

The term *Neuromuscular diseases yielded* 143 hits.

Creatinine phosphokinase activity
An early review by Meltzer (1976) dealt with the prevalence of an increased serum creatinine phospokinase activity (CPK) and with morphological changes in muscle fibres in psychiatric patients. He found increased prevalences in both serum CPK activity and abnormal muscle fibres and suggested that these results may show another organic component of the major psychoses, recommending

further research on a possible aetiological relation between neuromuscular dysfunction and schizophrenia.

3.10.14. Neurotoxicity syndromes

The term *Neurotoxicity syndromes* yielded 1482 hits. Most of the reports were on EPS of antipsychotic drugs, which have been briefly reviewed above (see subsection on movement disorders, p. 49).

3.10.15. Sleep disorders

The term *Sleep disorders* yielded 305 hits. Six reports were relevant (Benca *et al.* 1992, Kales and Marusak 1967, Monti and Monti 2004, Sweetwood *et al.* 1976, Takahashi *et al.* 1998). Since two comprehensive reviews were available, the following text focusses on their results (Benca *et al.* 1992, Monti and Monti 2004).

Sleep disturbances

Insomnia is a well-known symptom of schizophrenia which is often seen during exacerbations of schizophrenia and may precede the appearance of other symptoms of relapse (Monti and Monti 2004). A comprehensive meta-analysis including 177 studies with data from 7151 psychiatric patients and controls has been presented by Benca *et al.* (1992). A summary on schizophrenia showed that compared to other groups schizophrenics had altered sleep parameters on a variety of measures. Monti and Monti (2004) reviewed five studies ($n = 136$) on antipsychotic-drug-naïve patients with schizophrenia, and 13 controlled ($n = 390$) and nine uncontrolled ($n = 115$) studies on patients previously treated with neuroleptics. They concluded that sleep disturbances of either never-medicated or previously treated schizophrenia patients are characterized by a sleep-onset and maintenance insomnia. In addition, stage 4 sleep, slow-wave sleep (stages 3 and 4), non-REM sleep in minutes and REM latency are decreased.

Obstructive sleep apnoea

The study by Winkelman (2001) evaluated obstructive sleep apnoea (OSA) in schizophrenia. Since antipsychotics often cause weight gain (Allison *et al.* 1999b) and obesity is the most important risk factor for OSA (Young *et al.* 1993), obese psychiatric patients may be at risk for OSA. The sample consisted of 364 psychiatric patients, 46 of whom had schizophrenia. Obstructive sleep apnoea was defined as more than 20 instances of apnoea and/or hypapnoea per hour of sleep. Patients with schizophrenia/schizoaffective disorder were significantly heavier and had higher rates of OSA than patients with other psychiatric disorders. Obesity, male gender and chronic antipsychotic drug use were risk factors for OSA.

3.10.16. Trauma, nervous system

The term *Trauma, nervous system* yielded 190 hits. None was relevant.

3.11. Eye diseases

The MEDLINE search on *Eye Diseases* yielded 267 hits. From these 14 reports were ordered, and three of them were included. One report was added by cross-referencing.

3.11.1. Cataracts and hyperpigmentations of the lens and cornea

Ruigomez *et al.* (2000) investigated the incidence of cataracts in 4209 schizophrenic patients. The incidence rate of cataracts among schizophrenic patients (3.5 per 1000 person–years) was similar to that in the general population (4.5 per 1000 person–years). Antipsychotic drug use was not associated with the occurrence of cataracts; the relative risks were increased only in chlorpromazine and prochlorperazine users (8.8 and 4.0). There was no evidence that schizophrenia per se was associated with an increased risk of developing cataracts. While Ruigomez *et al.* (2000) had an epidemiological perspective, most of the other reports were on ocular side-effects of phenothiazines, especially chlorpromazine, which has been reported to cause hyperpigmentations of the lens and the cornea. Since this is a side-effect rather than a comorbid condition, details are not presented here.

3.11.2. Albinism

Clarke and Buckley (1989) reported two cases of familial coincidence of albinism and schizophrenia and hypothesized a common genetic linkage between the two disorders.

3.11.3. Blindness

The publication by Riscalla (1980) formulated a hypothesis that blindness may be a protective factor against schizophrenia.

In summary, with the exception of the side-effects of some old antipsychotic drugs, there is no evidence that schizophrenia is associated to a significant extent with eye diseases.

3.12. Urological and male genital diseases

The MEDLINE search on *Urologic and Male Genital Diseases* yielded 363 hits. Ten reports were ordered, of which six were included, and 18 reports were added by cross-referencing.

3.12.1. Urinary incontinence

Two reports were on urinary incontinence. Bonney *et al.* (1997) surveyed patients with schizophrenia and – as a comparison group – patients with mood disorder for urinary problems. Incontinence was more prevalent in schizophrenic patients than in the control group.

Lin *et al.* (1999) investigated the incidence of clozapine-associated urinary incontinence in schizophrenic patients. They found a transitory urinary incontinence in 44.3% of the patients and persistent urinary incontinence in 25% of these patients. They recommended monitoring every patient taking clozapine for the possibility of developing urinary incontinence.

3.12.2. Sexual dysfunction

Many studies report figures on antipsychotic-induced sexual dysfunction in patients with schizophrenia. An assessment of these medication effects would have gone beyond the scope of this review, because in theory this would have meant reviewing the entire antipsychotic drug literature. Since we were interested in the epidemiology of sexual dysfunction in schizophrenia, only studies that compared people with schizophrenia with non-schizophrenic controls were included and three such studies were identified:

Aizenberg *et al.* (1995) evaluated the sexual dysfunction of 20 untreated and 51 antipsychotic-treated male schizophrenic patients in comparison with 51 healthy controls. They used a detailed structured interview to assess sexual dysfunction quantitatively and qualitatively. Sexual dysfunction was reported in both groups of schizophrenic patients. Untreated schizophrenic patients exhibited mainly a decreased sexual desire whereas treated patients reported more impairments in erection and orgasm. The authors suggested that antipsychotic treatment is associated with restoration of sexual desire, but, on the other hand, that it can cause sexual dysfunction. They recommended that clinicians should be aware of these symptoms and openly discuss sexual problems with patients. This will improve comprehension and compliance.

Smith *et al.* (2002) developed a Sexual Functioning Questionnaire with detailed questions about libido, physical arousal (erection in men, vaginal lubrication in women), masturbation, orgasm (including dyspareunia) and ejaculation. They investigated 101 patients with conventional antipsychotic medication

Table 3.17. Cancer of the urinary system

Study	Country	Number of schizophrenic patients	Control group	Incidence rate for cancer of the urinary system in patients with schizophrenia
Mortensen 1989	Denmark	6152: men 2956, women 3196	General population of Denmark	IRR – men: 0.72 (s.), women: 1.26 (n.s.)
Mortensen 1994	Denmark	9156: men 5658, women 3498	General population of Denmark	SIR – men: 1.59 (n.s.), women: 1.13 (n.s.)
Goldacre *et al.* 2005	UK	9649	600 000 hospital patients in the Oxford Health Region	RR – 1.18 (n.s.)

IRR, incidence rate ratio (observed/expected number of cases standardized for age and sex); n.s., not statistically significant; RR, relative risk; s., statistically significant; SIR = standardized cancer incidence rate. RR, SIR, IRR < 1 = decreased incidence; RR, SIR, IRR > 1 = increased incidence.

and found a prevalence of 45% of sexual dysfunction. Of the 55 normal controls, sexual dysfunction occurred in 17%. Sexual dysfunction was associated with autonomic side-effects in normoprolactinaemic males, but the presence of hyperprolactinaemia overrode other causes of sexual dysfunction. For women, hyperprolactinaemia was the main cause of sexual dysfunction. Smith and colleagues recommended that clinicians should routinely enquire about sexual symptoms prior to the prescription of antipsychotics and on follow-up to prevent non-compliance in patients. Antipsychotics with fewer effects on prolactin should be used preferentially.

Macdonald *et al.* (2003) measured rates of sexual dysfunction in 135 people with schizophrenia in comparison with 114 healthy persons from the general population of Nithsdale, south-west Scotland. In a case-control design they assessed sexual dysfunction by a self-completed gender-specific questionnaire. People with schizophrenia reported much higher rates of sexual dysfunction than healthy controls: 82% of the men and 96% of the women reported at least one sexual dysfunction (healthy controls 38% and 58%). In female patients, sexual dysfunction was associated with negative symptoms and general psychopathology. There was no association between sexual dysfunction and type of antipsychotic medication.

In summary, sexual dysfunction appears to be a common problem in schizophrenic patients, but few studies provide epidemiological data. The causes appear to be intrinsic to schizophrenia on the one hand (e.g. negative symptoms) and medication related on the other hand. The relatively high rates of sexual

Table 3.18. Studies on the incidence of cancer of the urinary bladder in patients with schizophrenia

Study	Country	Number of schizophrenic patients	Control group	Incidence rate for lung cancer in patients with schizophrenia
Mortensen 1989	Denmark	6152: men 2956, women 3196	General population of Denmark	IRR – men: 0.66 (s.), women: 1.08 (n.s.)
Lawrence et al. 2000	Australia	172 932 patients with various psychiatric disorders (number of men and women unknown)	General population of Western Australia	RR – men: 1.03 (n.s.), women: 0.84 (n.s.)
Lichtermann et al. 2001	Finland	26 996	General population of Finland	SIR – 1.18 (n.s.)
Barak et al. 2005	Israel	3226	General Jewish population of Israel	SIR – 0.69 (n.s.)
Dalton et al. 2005	Denmark	22 766: men 13 023, women 9743	General population of Denmark	SIR – men: 0.78 (n.s.), women: 0.85 (n.s.)
Goldacre et al. 2005	UK	9649	600 000 hospital patients in the Oxford Health Region	RR – 0.79 (n.s.)

IRR, incidence rate ratio (observed/expected number of cases standardized for age and sex); n.s., not statistically significant; RR, relative risk; s., statistically significant; SIR, standardized cancer incidence rate. RR, SIR, IRR < 1 = decreased incidence; RR, SIR, IRR > 1 = increased incidence.

dysfunction in the healthy control groups of the included studies underline that controlled epidemiological studies are necessary to assess the true prevalence.

3.12.3. Cancers of the urinary system

Tables 3.17, 3.18 and 3.19 provide a summary of the prevalence of cancers of the urinary tract among schizophrenic patients that were derived from the population-based studies on cancer in the section on neoplasms (section 3.4). The data are heterogeneous, with most studies showing no statistically

Table 3.19. Cancer of the kidney

Study	Country	Number of schizophrenic patients	Control group	Incidence rate for cancer of the kidney in patients with schizophrenia
Mortensen 1989	Denmark	6152: men 2956, women 3196	General population of Denmark	IRR – men: 0.87 (n.s.), women: 1.46 (n.s.)
Lichtermann et al. 2001	Finland	26 996	General population of Finland	SIR – 1.30 (n.s.)
Barak et al. 2005	Israel	3226	General Jewish population of Israel	SIR – 1.09 (n.s.)
Dalton et al. 2005	Denmark	22 766: men: 13 023, women 9743	General population of Denmark	SIR – men: 1.00 (n.s.), women: 1.23 (n.s.)
Goldacre et al. 2005	UK	9649	600 000 hospital patients in the Oxford Health Region	RR – 0.95 (n.s.)

IRR, incidence rate ratio (observed/expected number of cases standardized for age and sex); n.s., not statistically significant; RR, relative risk; s., statistically significant; SIR, standardized cancer incidence rate. RR, SIR, IRR $< 1 =$ decreased incidence; RR, SIR, IRR $> 1 =$ increased incidence.

significant differences between groups. This research suffers from limited statistical power, and its results are inconclusive.

3.12.4. Prostate cancer

Results on the frequency of prostate cancer were derived from the section on neoplasms (section 3.4). The population-based studies reviewed there were analysed as to results on male forms of cancer. They consistently showed a decreased rate of prostate cancer in schizophrenia (see Table 3.20). Mortensen (1992) performed the only case-control study focussing specifically on the risk of prostate cancer in schizophrenic patients. In a nested case-control study of 38 cases and 76 age- and sex-matched controls, he found a decreased incidence of prostate cancer (incidence rate ratio $= 0.56$, $p < 0.01$). Those patients who had been treated with a cumulative dose of high-dose phenothiazines (primarily chlorpromazine) of 15 g or more had a reduced risk of prostate cancer. The patients had been treated with an average dose of 145 mg chlorpromazine

Table 3.20. Studies on the the incidence of prostate cancer in patients with schizophrenia

Study	Country	Number of male schizophrenic patients	Control group	Incidence rate for prostate cancer in patients with schizophrenia
Mortensen 1992	Denmark	2956	General population of Denmark	IRR – 0.56 (s.)
Lawrence et al. 2000	Australia	172 932 patients with various psychiatric disorders (number of men unknown)	General population of Western Australia	IRR – 0.87 (s.)
Lichtermann et al. 2001	Finland	15 578	General population of Finland	SIR – 0.49 (n.s.)
Barak et al. 2005	Israel	3226	General Jewish population of Israel	SIR – 0.31 (n.s.)
Dalton et al. 2005	Denmark	13 023	General population of Denmark	SIR – 0.56, (s.)
Goldacre et al. 2005	UK	9649 (number of men unknown)	600 000 individuals with various medical or surgical conditions	RR – 0.76 (n.s.)
Grinshpoon et al. 2005	Israel	26 518 (number of men unknown)	General population of Israel	SIR – 0.53 (s.)

IRR, incidence rate ratio (observed/expected number of cases standardized for age and sex); n.s., not statistically significant; RR, relative risk; s., statistically significant; SIR, standardized cancer incidence rate. RR, SIR, IRR < 1 = decreased incidence; RR, SIR, IRR > 1 = increased incidence.

for an average of 12.5 years. No other significant risk factors were identified. Mortensen suggested that antipsychotic drug treatment may be a protective factor. Phenothiazines have been found to have antiproliferative activity in vitro due to an antagonistic effect of calmodulin activity (Nordenberg et al. 1999), but convincing evidence in vivo is lacking. In a later report Mortensen (1994) suggested that the decreased risk of prostate cancer in some studies might be ascribed to reduced sexual activity (Rotkin 1977, Zaridze and Boyle 1987).

Table 3.21. Studies on the incidence of cancer of the testis in patients with schizophrenia

Study	Country	Number of male schizophrenic patients	Control group	Standardized incidence rate for testis cancer in patients with schizophrenia
Mortensen 1989	Denmark	2956	General population of Denmark	IRR – 0.39 (n.s.)
Barak *et al.* 2005	Israel	3226	General Jewish population of Israel	SIR – 0.47 (n.s.)
Dalton *et al.* 2005	Denmark	13 023	General population of Denmark	SIR – 0.69 (n.s.)
Goldacre *et al.* 2005	UK	9649 (number of men unknown)	600 000 individuals with various medical or surgical conditions	RR – 1.30 (n.s.)

IRR, incidence rate ratio (observed/expected number of cases standardized for age and sex); n.s., not statistically significant; RR, relative risk; SIR, standardized cancer incidence rate. RR, SIR, IRR < 1 = decreased incidence; RR, SIR, IRR > 1 = increased incidence.

3.12.5. Cancer of the testis

Only three studies investigated the risk for cancer of the testis, but none of them found a significant difference between groups (see Table 3.21).

3.13. Female genital diseases and pregnancy complications

The MEDLINE search on *Female Genital Diseases and Pregnancy Complications* yielded 554 hits. From these 34 reports were ordered, of which 14 were included; 23 reports were added by cross-referencing. Most of the studies were on obstetric or neonatal complications of offspring of parents with schizophrenia. Thirty relevant studies published between 1935 and 2005 were identified (see Table 3.22). Since this is an important area, first some important definitions in this area will be presented.

3.13.1. Obstetric and neonatal complications

Intrauterine growth retardation: deviation of intrauterine growth from the growth potential of the fetus. Birthweight below the 10th percentile for gestational age (Bennedsen 1998).

Preterm birth: delivery prior to 37 completed weeks of gestation (World Health Organization 1992).

Perinatal death: fetal death after 22 completed weeks of gestation or death before seven completed days after birth (World Health Organization 1992).

Stillbirth: fetal death occurring at the 28th gestational week or later (Nilsson *et al.* 2002).

Low birthweight: birthweight below 2500 g (World Health Organization 1992).

Low Apgar score: poor neonatal condition of the baby (Sacker *et al.* 1996). The Apgar score is that of the first test given to a newborn the first minute after birth and again at 5 minutes after birth and, in the event of serious problems with the baby's condition, at 10 minutes after birth. Five factors are evaluated and scored on a scale of 0 to 2: heart rate (pulse), breathing (rate and effort), activity and muscle tone, grimace response (reflex irritability) and appearance (skin coloration). Scores obtainable range between 10 and 0, with 10 being the highest possible score (Ural 2004).

Neonatal complications: defined as complications up to the 28th completed day of life (Webb *et al.* 2005).

Sudden infant death syndrome (SIDS): defined as the sudden death of a baby that is unexpected from the baby's history and unexplained by a thorough post-mortem examination (Hunt and Shannon 1992).

Infant death: death within the first year of life (Nilsson *et al.* 2002).

Table 3.22 shows that since the publication of the first study by Essen-Moller (1935), which in contrast to most later studies reported no difference in mortality risk between offspring of schizophrenic parents and the general population, many researchers have examined the pregnancy outcomes of patients with schizophrenia. Most studies investigated the specific effect of maternal schizophrenia, while only a few reports studied the effect of parental (mother and/or father afflicted) schizophrenia in general (Erlenmeyer-Kimling 1968, Essen-Moller W. 1935, Mednick *et al.* 1971, Modrzewska 1980, Rieder *et al.* 1975). The quality of the studies and the specific outcomes analysed varied substantially. However, some recent investigations (Bennedsen *et al.* 2001b, Jablensky *et al.* 2005, Nilsson *et al.* 2002) were population based using national registries allowing generalization.

Most studies did find increased rates of obstetric complications among mothers with schizophrenia, although there are a few exceptions and some effects in the reverse direction. For example, while the population-based study by Bennedsen *et al.* (2001a) found increased rates of birth complications in general among mothers with schizophrenia, the rate of pre-eclampsia was reduced (Bennedsen *et al.* 2001b) – a finding that the authors explain by the increased rates of smokers among schizophrenic mothers, because smoking has been shown to reduce the risk of pre-eclampsia (Cnattingius *et al.* 1997, Sibai *et al.* 1995). Nevertheless,

Table 3.22. Obstetric complications in schizophrenic women and neonatal complications in offspring of schizophrenic parents

Study	Country	Study period	Research question	Number of mothers with schizophrenia (MS), children of mothers with schizophrenia (CMS) and parents with schizophrenia (PS); control groups: mothers (CM), children (CC) and parents (CP) without schizophrenia	Pregnancy complications (PC), obstetric complications (OC), neonatal complications (NC)	Data source on schizophrenia and maternal and child health	Conclusions
Essen-Moller 1935	Germany		Mortality in offspring of male parents with schizophrenia in Munich	Not available	Not available	Not available	No evidence or difference in risk of mortality for offspring with exposure to parental schizophrenia
Wiedorn 1954	USA		Prevalence of toxaemia (blood pressure of 140/90 mm HG or above, together with albuminuria or oedema in the last trimester) in schizophrenic women compared to women without psychotic disorder	MS: 72 CM: 54 Number of pregnancies of schizophrenic women: 155 Number of pregnancies of normal women: 155	Toxaemia: 46.4% vs. 22.2%	Case records from the Charity Hospital of New Orleans	Higher incidence of toxaemia of pregnancy in schizophrenic women

Study	Country	Years	Aims/methods	Sample	Results	Data source	Conclusions
Paffenberger et al. 1961	USA	1940–58	(1) Prevalence of obstetric complications of women between 15 and 44 years who had their first psychotic attack 6 months before or after childbirth in the Cincinnati, Ohio, hospital service area. Control group were women matched on race without psychosis who delivered at the same obstetric unit (2) Prevalence of perinatal mortality	Psychotic mothers: 126 (57 with schizophrenia) CM: 252	OC: Pre-eclampsia: 7% vs. 5% NC: Fetal death or neonatal death: 6% vs. 3%	Medical charts of all hospitals with psychiatric services and hospital obstetric records of each psychotic subject. County or state tabulations by the Ohio Department of Health	Larger proportions of psychotic patients manifested pre-eclampsia during pregnancy. The perinatal mortality rate was higher among infants of psychotic patients.

Table 3.22. (cont.)

Study	Country	Study period	Research question	Number of mothers with schizophrenia (MS), children of mothers with schizophrenia (CMS) and parents with schizophrenia (PS); control groups: mothers (CM), children (CC) and parents (CP) without schizophrenia	Pregnancy complications (PC), obstetric complications (OC), neonatal complications (NC)	Data source on schizophrenia and maternal and child health	Conclusions
Sobel 1961	USA	1950–8	Prevalence of stillbirth, neonatal death and congenital malformations in offspring of maternal schizophrenia. Comparison with the rate in the general population (US National Office of Vital Statistics 1950)	MS: 218 CM: general population CMS: 222 CC: Newborn in the general population	NC: 8.1% vs. 3.6% Congenital malformations: 3.2% vs. 0.8%	Delivery records from seven New York state mental hospitals	Twofold higher risk of perinatal death, threefold higher risk of congenital malformations in offspring of maternal schizophrenia

Erlenmeyer-Kimling 1968	USA	1900–59	Infant mortality and deaths to age 15 years in the offspring of parental schizophrenia. Comparison with US birth cohorts of the same decades	PS: 691 CP: general population CMS: 1718 CC: general population	NC: 109 deaths Medical records and infant and childhood survival rates from state hospitals in New York	Compared with the rates in the general population there was lower infant mortality (30% lower in males and 60% lower in females) during the first year of life in the offspring of schizophrenic parents
Lane and Albee 1970	USA		Comparison of birthweights of children born to schizophrenic women and born to women without a psychotic disorder	MS: 281 CM: 281	Mean birthweight: 3116 g vs. 3127 g Hospital records	Slightly lower birthweight in offspring of schizophrenic women

Table 3.22. (*cont.*)

Study	Country	Study period	Research question	Number of mothers with schizophrenia (MS), children of mothers with schizophrenia (CMS) and parents with schizophrenia (PS); control groups: mothers (CM), children (CC) and parents (CP) without schizophrenia	Pregnancy complications (PC), obstetric complications (OC), neonatal complications (NC)	Data source on schizophrenia and maternal and child health	Conclusions
Mednick *et al.* 1971	Denmark	1959–61	Perinatal conditions in children of schizophrenic parents. Comparison with normal parents who delivered also in the University Hospital in Copenhagen	PS: 83 (42 men, 41 women) CP: 83	Mean birthweight: 3054 vs. 3263 g	Danish Central Psychiatric Registry Records of the Bispebjerg Hospital in Copenhagen, delivery records from the University Hospital in Copenhagen	Mildly lower birthweight among children born to schizophrenic parents. Female infants suffered more from pregnancy complications, especially if the father was schizophrenic
Sameroff and Zax 1973	USA		Prevalence of delivery complications in schizophrenic mothers and abnormal EEGs in offspring of schizophrenic mothers, compared with mothers without psychopathology	MS: 12 CM: 13 CMS: 12 CC: 12	OC: Delivery complications: 3 vs. 9 NC: Abnormal EEG: 6 vs. 3	Monroe County Psychiatric Register Delivery protocols from the Strong Memorial Hospital, Rochester, NY	Higher proportion of abnormal EEGs in the offspring of schizophrenic mothers

68

Study	Country/Year	Aim	Sample	Source	Results	Conclusions
McNeil and Kaij 1973	Sweden	Obstetric complications in offspring of schizophrenic mothers compared to offspring of normal mothers	MS: 32 CM: 32	Swedish Population Register Hospital records from the state Psychiatric Hospital in Malm and the Malm General Hospital	PC: 0.59% vs. 0.44% OC: 0.88% vs. 0.63% Mean all disturbances: 2.28% vs. 1.75% Mean birthweight: 3409 g vs. 3538 g	No significant differences in the rates of pregnancy, birth and placental complications between schizophrenic mothers and their controls. No significant differences in gestational age, birthweight, body length, head and shoulder circumference.
Mirdal et al. 1974	Denmark 1962–3	Prevalence of PBCs in children of schizophrenic mothers compared to mothers without a history of hospitalization for mental illness	MS: 112 CM: 84 CMS: 166 CC: 90	Midwife protocols	OC: Total PBC rate: 2.79% vs. 2.51% Severe PBCs: 11.5% vs. 7.8% Mean number of PBCs: 1.43 vs. 1.29 NC: Mean birthweight: 3449 g vs. 3395 g	No significant differences in the number or severity of PBCs between the two groups. However, significantly higher rates of PBCs among first pregnancies and deliveries of schizophrenic women as

Table 3.22. (*cont.*)

Study	Country	Study period	Research question	Number of mothers with schizophrenia (MS), children of mothers with schizophrenia (CMS) and parents with schizophrenia (PS); control groups: mothers (CM), children (CC) and parents (CP) without schizophrenia	Pregnancy complications (PC), obstetric complications (OC), neonatal complications (NC)	Data source on schizophrenia and maternal and child health	Conclusions
							compared to the first reproductions of normal women. Normal women tended to have higher rates of PBCs with increasing age and parity, whereas neither age nor delivery number affected the rate of PBCs among schizophrenic mothers

Study	Country	Aim	Sample	Results	Method	Conclusion
Cohler et al. 1975	USA	Prevalence of pregnancy and birth complications among schizophrenic and well mothers and their children	MS: 28 CM: 44	OC: Pregnancy and birth complications: 37% vs. 22% NC: Lower birthweight: 5.9% vs. 5.7%	Data from discharge records from a psychiatric hospital in the greater Boston area; the matched control sample was recruited by means of newspaper advertisements	More PBCs among women with acute rather than chronic disturbance
Ragins et al. 1975	USA	Prevalence of low birthweight, pregnancy and birth complications and low Apgar scores in offspring of schizophrenic mothers	MS: 14 CM: 18	Mean birthweight: 6.9 pounds (3133 g) vs. 7.7 pounds (3496 g) PBCs: 50% vs. 50% Apgar score <8: 21.43% vs. 16.67%	All pregnant women who came for prenatal care to a large, urban, university-affiliated obstetric and gynaecological hospital; psychiatric screening questionnaire	Lower birthweights and lower Apgar scores among offspring of schizophrenic mothers. No difference in pregnancy and birth complications between schizophrenic mothers and controls

Table 3.22. (cont.)

Study	Country	Study period	Research question	Number of mothers with schizophrenia (MS), children of mothers with schizophrenia (CMS) and parents with schizophrenia (PS); control groups: mothers (CM), children (CC) and parents (CP) without schizophrenia	Pregnancy complications (PC), obstetric complications (OC), neonatal complications (NC)	Conclusions
Rieder et al. 1975	USA		Fetal death and neonatal death in offspring of parental schizophrenia spectrum disorders,[a] matched controls without a diagnosis of schizophrenia were taken from the same sample	CMS: 93 CC: 186	NC: Fetal and neonatal deaths: 7.5% vs. 3.8% Mean birthweight: 3335 g vs. 3341 g	Data source on schizophrenia and maternal and child health Data from the Perinatal Research Branch of the National Institute of Neurological Diseases and Stroke (NINDS) in cooperation with 12 university-affiliated hospitals; the Boston subgroup was chosen as sample	Non-significantly higher risk of fetal and neonatal death in offspring of parents with schizophrenia

Reference	Country	Aim	Sample	Results	Source	Conclusion
Rieder et al. 1977	USA	Comparison of Apgar scores between offspring of schizophrenic parents and normal controls and prevalence of obstetric complications in schizophrenic mothers	CMS: 60 CC: 60	Mean Apgar score: 8.65 vs. 8.875 OC: Swelling in pregnancy: 31.18% vs. 30.35% Vaginal bleeding: 46.38% vs. 42.03% Hypertension/proteinuria: 13.13% vs. 10.35%	Perinatal Research Branch of the Boston National Institute of Neurological and Communicative Disorders and Stroke (NINCDS); hospital records	Lower Apgar scores among offspring of schizophrenic parents and higher rates of obstetric complications in schizophrenic women
Zax et al. 1977	USA	Birth outcomes in the offspring of mentally disordered women with different psychiatric diagnoses compared to a normal control group	MS: 29 CM: 80	NC: Low birthweight: 0.14% vs. 0.0%	Monroe County Hospital psychiatric register records of all women who delivered at a local hospital in Monroe County since 1959	Lighter birthweight in schizophrenic women's offspring

Table 3.22. (*cont.*)

Study	Country	Study period	Research question	Number of mothers with schizophrenia (MS), children of mothers with schizophrenia (CMS) and parents with schizophrenia (PS); control groups: mothers (CM), children (CC) and parents (CP) without schizophrenia	Pregnancy complications (PC), obstetric complications (OC), neonatal complications (NC)	Data source on schizophrenia and maternal and child health	Conclusions
Modrzewska 1980	Sweden	1946–9, 1972–7	Prevalence of stillbirth and infant death in offspring of 214 known schizophrenic patients born between 1829 and 1960 in a North Swedish isolate compared with children of unaffected parents in the same population.	CMS: 553 CC: 624	NC: Stillbirths: 3.4% vs. 1.1% Infant mortality: 4.7% vs.1.1%	Parish registers from a North Swedish isolate (three parishes: Pajala, Muonionalusta, Junosuando)	Threefold higher risk of stillbirth, fourfold higher risk of infant death

Study	Country	Years	Aim	Sample	Results	Data source	Conclusion
Wrede et al. 1980	Finland	1960–4	Prevalence of pregnancy complications and delivery complications in the births of Finnish children with schizophrenic mothers; controls without schizophrenia were chosen by taking the hospital delivery immediately preceding that of the index child	MS: 171 (54 chronic and 117 mild schizophrenic mothers) CM: 171	PC: first trimester: chronic: 31.8%, mild: 9.6% vs. 17% (controls); second trimester: chronic: 22.7%, mild: 14.9% vs. 15.9% (controls); third trimester: chronic: 46.8%, mild: 26.6% vs. 17.8% (controls) OC: moderate complications: chronic: 19.6%, mild: 21.2% vs. 22.3%; severe complications: chronic: 15.7%, mild: 24.8% vs. 9.1%	Finnish perinatal Care System Population Register of the city of Helsinki Well Mother–Baby Clinic records	Higher rates of pregnancy complications in chronic schizophrenic mothers, especially significant in the first and third trimester; significantly higher rates of severe delivery complications in schizophrenic mothers

Table 3.22. (*cont.*)

Study	Country	Study period	Research question	Number of mothers with schizophrenia (MS), children of mothers with schizophrenia (CMS) and parents with schizophrenia (PS); control groups: mothers (CM), children (CC) and parents (CP) without schizophrenia	Pregnancy complications (PC), obstetric complications (OC), neonatal complications (NC)	Data source on schizophrenia and maternal and child health	Conclusions
Marcus et al. 1981	USA	1973–7	Comparison of birthweights of children born to schizophrenic parents and children born to parents without a psychotic disorder	PS: 17 CP: 18	Birthweight: 2982 g vs. 3180 g	Chart records of Maternal and Child Care Centres of the Municipality of Jerusalem and interviews and questionnaires about pregnancy	Low to low–normal birthweights in offspring of schizophrenic parents
Shinmoto et al. 1989	Japan	1983–8	Prevalence of pregnancy complications in schizophrenic women, comparison with deliveries of normal women in the Saga Medical School	MS: 7 CM: 1458	OC: 6 Caesarean section: 3 No control data.	Delivery records from the Saga Medical School	Six out of seven cases grew worse during their pregnancies. Three women underwent Caesarean section due to their mental illness

Study	Country	Years	Objective	Scores	Results	Sample	Findings
Goodman and Emory 1992	USA		Prevalence of pregnancy and birth complications in births to schizophrenic women, comparison with control sample from well-baby clinics in the same neighbourhood	MS: 57 CM: 31	NC: Mean birthweight: 3000 g vs. 3211 g Mean Apgar score 5 min: 8.78 vs. 8.96	Patient sample from inner-city outpatient clinics (93% were African-American)	Schizophrenic mothers, especially older ones, had significantly smaller babies with lower Apgar scores and had more pregnancy and birth complications overall
Miller and Finnerty 1996	USA	1993–5	Prevalence of obstetric complications in schizophrenic mothers and prevalence of stillbirth in offspring of maternal schizophrenia; comparison with subjects without major mental illness who were matched for age, race, education, employment status and religion	MS: 46 CM: 50	OC: 54.3% vs. 66% NC: Stillbirth: 5.6% vs. 6.5%	Patient and control group recruited from in- and outpatient medical and psychiatric services affiliated with a teaching hospital serving a geographically, economically and culturally diverse population	No evident difference in risk of obstetrical complications and stillbirth between schizophrenia patients and controls

Table 3.22. (cont.)

Study	Country	Study period	Research question	Number of mothers with schizophrenia (MS), children of mothers with schizophrenia (CMS) and parents with schizophrenia (PS); control groups: mothers (CM), children (CM) and parents (CC) and parents (CP) without schizophrenia	Pregnancy complications (PC), obstetric complications (OC), neonatal complications (NC)	Data source on schizophrenia and maternal and child health	Conclusions
Schubert *et al.* 1996	Sweden		Comparison of wakefulness and arousal in neonates born to women with schizophrenia and neonates born to women with no history of psychosis	MS: 20 CM: 25	NC: Reduced wakefulness: 35% *vs.* 8%	Sample from a longitudinal high-risk study in southern Sweden (McNeil *et al.* 1983)	The offspring of mothers with schizophrenia had significantly reduced arousal as compared with their control cases
Bennedsen *et al.* 1999	Denmark	1973–93	Prevalence of preterm birth, low birthweight and intrauterine growth retardation among children of women with schizophrenia; comparison with a 10% random sample of all live births during 1973–1993 of birth-giving women in Denmark	MS:1537 CM: 727 42 CMS: 2212 CC: 122 931	NC: Preterm birth: 6.9% *vs.* 4.5% Birthweight (mean): males: 3335 g *vs.* 3472 g, females: 3245 g *vs.* 3357 g Intrauterine growth retardation: 14.7% *vs.* 10.3%	Danish Psychiatric Case Register, Danish Medical Birth Register	The children of women with schizophrenia were at increased risk of preterm delivery, low birthweight and small for gestational age

Study	Country	Years	Aim	Sample	Results	Conclusions
Preti *et al.* 2000	Italy	1964–78	Prevalence of obstetric complications in schizophrenic women and prevalence of pre- or perinatal complications in the offspring of schizophrenic mothers; comparison with normal healthy control subjects matched by maternal age and marital status and by gender, time and parity of birth	MS: 44 CM: 44 CMS: 44 CC: 44	44 case-control subjects born between 1964 and 1978 in Padova, Italy	OC: 75% vs. 59% (OR: 2.07) OC with clear damaging potential: 34% vs. 9% OC among males vs. females: 41% vs. 15% Complications per birth: 2:1 Miscarriages MS: OR 4.66 Preterm births MS: OR 2.58 NC: Gestational age: no difference Birthweight: no difference	Severe, brain-damaging obstetric complications would seem to be a possible antecedent of a diagnosis of schizophrenia or a related disorder in adulthood. Some early-onset cases may be accounted for by prenatal brain lesions. This enhanced risk of negative pregnancy outcome may be under genetic control, contributing to the persistence of schizophrenia in the general population

Table 3.22. (cont.)

Study	Country	Study period	Research question	Number of mothers with schizophrenia (MS), children of mothers with schizophrenia (CMS) and parents with schizophrenia (PS); control groups: mothers (CM), children (CM), children (CC) and parents (CP) without schizophrenia	Pregnancy complications (PC), obstetric complications (OC), neonatal complications (NC)	Data source on schizophrenia and maternal and child health	Conclusions
Bennedsen et al. 2001b	Denmark	1973–93	Prevalence of obstetric complications in women with schizophrenia; comparison with a 10% random sample of all live births during 1973–1993 of birth-giving women in Denmark	MS: 1537 CM: 72 742 CS: 2212 CC: 122 931	OC: Relative risk for pre-eclampsia: 0.44% (s.)	Danish Psychiatric Case Register, Danish Medical Birth Register	Statistically significantly lower risk of pre-eclampsia in schizophrenic women. There was no other statistically significant difference in the risk of 13 others specific complications. Nevertheless, they were at increased risk for interventions during delivery

	Country	Years	Description	Numbers	Results	Data source	Conclusions
Bennedsen et al. 2001a	Denmark	1973–93 1983–92	(1) Prevalence of stillbirth, neonatal and postneonatal death in offspring of maternal schizophrenia. The control group were all women who gave birth to a single child in Denmark on 1 to 3 randomly selected days each month (2) Prevalence of congenital malformations in offspring of maternal schizophrenia; same control group as in (1)	(1) Risk for stillbirth and infant death: CMS: 2230 CC: 123 544 (2) Risk for congenital malformations: CMS: 746 CC: 56 106	NC: Adjusted relative risk for (1) Stillbirth: 1.63% vs. 0.5% (n.s.) Neonatal death: 1.26% vs. 0.5% (n.s.) Postneonatal death: 2.76% vs. 0.3% (s.) SIDS: 5.23% vs. 0.1% (s.) (2) Congenital malformations: 1.70% vs. 1.2% (s.)	Danish Psychiatric Central Register, Danish Medical Birth Registry, Danish National Registry of Congenital Malformations	Higher risk of stillbirth and postneonatal death, almost fivefold higher risk of SIDS, higher risk of congenital malformations in children from schizophrenic mothers
Nilsson et al. 2002	Sweden	1983–97	Prevalence of stillbirth and infant death in offspring of maternal schizophrenia; comparison with births in the general population	CS: 2096 CC: 1 555 975	NC: Stillbirth rate: 7.2/1000 births vs. 3.4/1000 Infant death rates: 11.9/1000 births vs. 4.9/1000	Medical Birth Register of Sweden, Swedish Inpatient Register	Twofold higher risk of stillbirth and infant death, additional excess risk if the mother was first admitted during pregnancy

Table 3.22. (*cont.*)

Study	Country	Study period	Research question	Number of mothers with schizophrenia (MS), children of mothers with schizophrenia (CMS) and parents with schizophrenia (PS); control groups: mothers (CM), children (CC) and parents (CP) without schizophrenia	Pregnancy complications (PC), obstetric complications (OC), neonatal complications (NC)	Data source on schizophrenia and maternal and child health	Conclusions
Howard *et al.* 2003	UK	1996–8	Prevalence of stillbirth and neonatal death in offspring of maternal psychotic disorders; comparison with women with no history of psychosis who had had children during the same years, matched for age and general practice	Mothers: 199 with psychotic disorder (34 with schizophrenia) CM: 787	OC: Caesarean sections: 20% vs. 14% NC: Stillbirths: 2.5% vs. <1% Neonatal deaths: 2% vs. 0%	General Practice Research Database	No significant difference in the risk of most individual obstetric complications. However, there were more Caesarean sections among women with psychotic disorders. Not significantly higher risk of stillbirth, significantly higher risk of neonatal death in women with psychotic disorders
Dickerson *et al.* 2004	USA	Mar–Dec 2000	Study on sexual and reproductive behaviour of women and men with a major	MS: 73 CM: 1145	NC: Stillbirth: 63% vs. 44%	Two outpatient psychiatric centres in the Baltimore Region Third	Women with mental illness had fewer pregnancies and live births, but were more

Study	Country	Period	Aim	Sample size	Results	Data source	Conclusions
			mental disorder or schizophrenia compared with those of persons from a national health survey matched for age and race			National Health and Examination Survey (NHANES III)	likely to have had a pregnancy that did not result in a live birth
Jablensky et al. 2005	Australia	1980–92	Prevalence of pregnancy, delivery and neonatal complications in a population cohort of women with schizophrenia who gave birth in Western Australia; comparison with births of women without a psychiatric diagnosis	MS: 328 CM: 1831 CMS: 618 CC: 3129	PC: 33.2% vs. 25.6% OC: 47.6% vs. 46.7% NC: 36.9% vs. 31.5%	Mental Health Information System of Western Australia Maternal and Child Health Research Database	Increased risk of pregnancy, birth and neonatal complications including placental abnormalities, antepartum haemorrhages and fetal disorders in schizophrenic patients. Significantly increased risk of placental abruption, low weight infants, children with cardiovascular abnormalities in women with schizophrenia

EEG, electroencephalogram; n.s., not statistically significant; OR, odds ratio; PBCs, pregnancy and birth complications; s., statistically significant; SIDS, sudden infant death syndrome.

[a] Includes offspring with exposure to parental schizophrenia ($n = 93$), possible schizophrenia/schizophrenic spectrum ($n = 60$) and others disorders ($n = 57$).

Source: Adapted from Sacker *et al.* (1996) and Webb *et al.* (2005) and completed by our MEDLINE search.

a recent meta-analysis focussing on mortality in offspring (Webb *et al.* 2005) also concluded that the risk of obstetric complications is increased.

Despite this widely accepted finding, there is a debate on the reasons underlying the increased risk, study designs and open questions in the area.

Possible reasons for the increased risk are shown in Table 3.23. It is quite plausible that the nature of schizophrenia leads to pregnancies and births that are mentally, behaviourally and socially complicated. Many women with schizophrenia are smokers and it may be more difficult for them to stop smoking or drinking alcohol during pregnancy (Jeste *et al.* 1996). They must take antipsychotic medication and may even take illicit drugs. All these factors may well contribute to adverse pregnancy outcomes. The disturbed state of mind in schizophrenia also troubles the experience of pregnancy, and it is likely that many women are not able to take care of themselves and their babies. They do not recognize comorbid medical conditions and tend to have lower attendance at antenatal care clinics (Bagedahl-Strindlund 1986, Bennedsen *et al.* 2001b, Kelly and McCreadie 1999, Wrede *et al.* 1980). These factors, together with low socioeconomic status, may well explain the observed increased risk of bad pregnancy outcome. There are also discussions on genetic factors, but there is no compelling evidence for such hypotheses yet.

Among many methodological problems in this research field, e.g. often imprecise definitions of the outcomes measured, varying definitions of schizophrenia, insufficient control for confounders (Bennedsen 1998), two fundamental issues have been stressed (Webb *et al.* 2005): (1) most studies were not population based and (2) they lacked sufficiently large sample sizes. Important open questions in the field are whether the risk is also increased when only the father has schizophrenia and whether the risk is higher if both parents are mentally ill. Are there gender differences between male and female offspring in terms of risk? Which of the risk factors summarized above are the most severe ones? Is the risk also increased in mental disorders other than schizophrenia, for example in bipolar disorder? Finally, very little is known about the effectiveness of specific interventions such as the separation of birth parent(s) (Webb *et al.* 2005).

In summary, there is sufficient evidence that schizophrenic women have more obstetric complications than normal controls, and it appears logical that the severe nature of schizophrenia explains a substantial part of this increased risk. Increased psychiatric and medical attention during the pregnancies of schizophrenic women and the improvement of preventive strategies in antenatal and postnatal care is needed. This need is underlined by the well-known association of adverse pregnancy outcome and the later development of schizophrenia in afflicted children (Kunugi *et al.* 2001).

3.13.2. Galactorrhoea

Counter to expectations, the search on *Female genital diseases and pregnancy complications* revealed very few epidemiological studies of the prevalence of

Table 3.23. Factors that may contribute to the association between schizophrenia and obstetric complications

Environmental factors	Pharmacological factors	Other factors
Toxic exposures	Psychotropic drugs	Psychological factors
Smoking		Maternal stress (life events, well-being,
Alcohol		attitude towards pregnancy, social
Cannabinoids		support)
Cocaine		Genetic predisposition and constitutional
Caffeine		factors
Socioeconomic		Maternal age
factors		Obstetric factors (nulliparity, multiparity,
Income		history of previous obstetric
Education		complications)
Marital status		Nutritional factors
Social class		Maternal physical illness (chronic diseases,
		genital or urinary tract infections)
		Antenatal care

Source: Adapted from Bennedsen (1998).

galactorrhoea and amenorrhoea. We found one study (Windgassen *et al.* 1996) on galactorrhoea in *Diseases of the nervous system* and added eight studies by cross-referencing.

Many antipsychotic drugs increase prolactin, which stimulates breast tissue growth and differentiation and lactation. It is well known that antipsychotic medication can therefore cause galactorrhoea (lactation) in both men and women. For example, Kleinberg *et al.* (1999) reported a 1.5% prevalence of galactorrhoea in women treated with risperidone and a 3.3% prevalence in women treated with haloperidol in pivotal risperidone studies. However, randomized controlled drug trials are likely to underestimate the risk of galactorrhoea, because they use patient interviews. The majority of the patients may not report their symptoms, because they experience it as something very personal and intimate (Wesselmann and Windgassen 1995). Therefore, studies with the aim of specifically assessing galactorrhoea from an epidemiological point of view would be more appropriate. Probably the best study, that by Windgassen *et al.* (1996), assessed the frequency of galactorrhoea in 150 schizophrenic patients, all of whom were treated with typical antipsychotics. The incidence between the 7th and the 75th day after the start of antipsychotic therapy was 14% and the prevalence 19%. The mean prolactin value for these patients was 55 ng/ml, but four patients with galactorrhoea had prolactin levels within the normal range. Previous pregnancies, premenopausal status and antipsychotic dose were significantly associated with the risk of galactorrhoea. In other studies that were in part reviewed by Windgassen *et al.* (1996) the frequency of galactorrhoea ranged between 10% and 57% (Apostolakis and Kapetanakis 1972, Davis and Cole 1975, Inoue *et al.* 1980, Neimeier *et al.* 1959, Py and Mathieu 1960, Turkington 1972, Wesselmann and Windgassen 1995, Zito *et al.* 1990). It is likely that the divergent rates can be explained by different sample compositions, different medication, different examination methods (use of milk pumps, manual examination, interviewing of patients) and inconsistent definitions of galactorrhoea.

Further epidemiologic studies on the occurrence of galactorrhoea in people with schizophrenia treated with atypical antipsychotics other than risperidone and amisulpride are needed, because there is a hope that their rates of galactorrhoea would be much lower.

3.13.3. Amenorrhoea

Since again the original search did not identify articles on amenorrhoea, a specific MEDLINE search was carried out that yielded 57 hits, none of which were relevant. The studies quoted below were thus taken from *Musculoskeletal Diseases* or added by cross-referencing. The ovarian function is regulated by the release of luteinizing hormone (LH) and follicle-stimulating hormone (FSH) which are regulated by the gonadotropin-releasing hormone (GRH). High prolactin levels induced by antipsychotic drugs can inhibit the hypothalamic release of GRH and this can lead to a disrupted ovarian function including irregular menses, dysmenorrhoea and even amenorrhoea. However, some studies showed that prolactin per se is not associated with likelihood of irregular menses (Canuso *et al.* 2002, Kleinberg *et al.* 1999, Magharious *et al.* 1998, Perkins 2003).

The prevalence of irregular menses or amenorrhoea has been reported as between 18.8% and 78% in women treated with typical antipsychotics (Beaumont and Dimond 1973, Ghadirian *et al.* 1982, Gingell *et al.* 1993, Inoue *et al.* 1980, Perkins 2003, Sandison *et al.* 1960, Shader and Grinspoon 1970). It has been reported that menstrual cycle abnormalities were associated with schizophrenia even in women with schizophrenia who had never been treated with antipsychotic medications. Considering the high prevalence of amenorrhoea and the clinical importance of a chronic low oestrogen state on cardiovascular health and osteoporosis (Grady *et al.* 1992), further research is needed (Perkins 2003).

3.13.4. Breast cancer

Studies on breast cancer derived from the MEDLINE search on *Neoplasms* and complemented by cross-referencing are summarized below.

A general question is whether high prolactin levels really promote breast cancer. While some authors support this view (Goffin *et al.* 1999, Llovera *et al.* 2000), according to others the epidemiological evidence is inconsistent (Bernstein and Ross 1993, Clevenger *et al.* 2003), with some studies showing a positive association (Ingram *et al.* 1990, Rose and Pruitt 1981) but others not (Bernstein *et al.* 1990, Secreto *et al.* 1983).

The results of the population-based studies on the relationship between schizophrenia and breast cancer are also inconclusive. Only two studies showed a statistically significantly increased risk of breast cancer in schizophrenia (Dalton *et al.* 2005, Nakane and Ohta 1986), while the other studies showed no significant differences (see Table 3.24).

3.13.5. Cancer of the cervix uteri

Data on cancer of the cervix uteri were again heterogeneous (see Table 3.25). Mortensen (1994) suggested that reduced sexual activity of people with schizophrenia (Rotkin 1977, Zaridze and Boyle 1987) might account for the reduced risk found in some studies, although this was statistically significant only in Dupont *et al.* (1986).

3.13.6. Cancer of the corpus uteri

The results on cancer of the corpus uteri were heterogeneous (see Table 3.26). While two studies showed a statistically significantly increased risk (Grinshpoon *et al.* 2005, Lichtermann *et al.* 2001), the other studies showed no significant differences compared to the general population, some of them even showing a trend towards decreased risk.

3.13.7. Cancer of the ovary

Finally, the results from studies on the risk for cancer of the ovary were again inconsistent, but no study showed statistically significant between-group differences (see Table 3.27). Definitive evidence is not available for any type of female cancers. A general problem with this research is that many studies were underpowered. They may have been sufficiently large to make a judgement about cancer in general, but not on specific cancers occurring more seldom.

3.14. Cardiovascular diseases

The MEDLINE search on *Cardiovascular Diseases* yielded 568 hits. From these 18 reports were ordered, 16 were included and eight reports were added by cross-referencing.

First, some important definitions and established facts from general medicine are provided:

Cardiovascular risk factors: established risk factors are age, male sex, smoking status, diabetic status, blood pressure, cholesterol/lipid concentrations

Table 3.24. Population-based studies on the association between schizophrenia and breast cancer

Study	Country	Number of female schizophrenic patients	Control group	Incidence rate for breast cancer in patients with schizophrenia
Nakane and Ohta 1986	Japan	1388	General population of Nagasaki city	RR: 3.2 (s.) Women born after 1925: 8.06 (s.)
Mortensen 1989	Denmark	2956 men, 3196 women	General population of Denmark	IRR: men: 1.85 (n.s.), women: 1.19 (n.s.)
Gulbinat et al. 1992	USA (Hawaii)	2779	1195 with affective psychosis, 142 with paranoid psychoses, 43 888 with other conditions	RR: Honolulu: Japanese women: 1.60 (n.s.)
Mortensen 1994	Denmark	5658 men, 3498 women	General population of Denmark	SIR: men: 0.00 (n.s.), women: 0.88 (n.s.)
Halbreich and Palter 1996	USA	275 female psychiatric patients	928 age-matched women without a psychiatric disorder	Schizophrenic women: 3.5 times higher risk than in normal controls
Lawrence et al. 2000	Australia	172 932 patients with various psychiatric disorders (number of women unknown)	General population of Western Australia	IRR: women: 0.98 (n.s.)

Study	Country	Number	Comparison population	Result
Lichtermann et al. 2001	Finland	11 418	General population of Finland	SIR: women: 1.15 (n.s.)
Dalton et al. 2003	Denmark	7541	13 28 772 women of the general population	RR: Women: 0.91 (n.s.)
Barak et al. 2005	Israel	3226	General Jewish population of Israel	SIR: 0.61 (s.)
Dalton et al. 2005	Denmark	9743	General population of Denmark	SIR: women: 1.20 (s.), men: 1.00 (n.s.)
Goldacre et al. 2005	UK	9649 (number of women unknown)	600 000 individuals with various medical or surgical conditions	RR: 1.01 (n.s.)
Grinshpoon et al. 2005	Israel	26 518 (number of women unknown)	General population of Israel	SIR: women: 1.11 (n.s.)

IRR, incidence rate ratio (observed/expected number of cases standardized for age and sex); n.s., not statistically significant; RR, relative risk; s., statistically significant; SIR, standardized cancer incidence rate. RR, SIR, IRR < 1 = decreased incidence; RR, SIR, IRR > 1 = increased incidence.

Table 3.25. Population-based studies on the association between schizophrenia and cancer of the cervix uteri

Study	Country	Number of female schizophrenic patients	Control group	Incidence rate for cancer of the cervix uteri in patients with schizophrenia
Mortensen 1989	Denmark	3196	General population of Denmark	IRR: 0.68 (n.s.)
Gulbinat et al. 1992	(USA) (Hawaii)	2779	1195 with affective psychosis, 142 with paranoid psychoses, 43 888 with other conditions	RR: Honolulu Japanese women: 3.25 (n.s.)
Lawrence et al. 2000	Australia	172 932 patients with various psychiatric disorders (number of women unknown)	General population of Western Australia	IRR: 1.02 (n.s.)
Lichtermann et al. 2001	Finland	11 418	General population of Finland	SIR: 1.31 (n.s.)
Barak et al. 2005	Israel	3226	General Jewish population of Israel	SIR: 0.58 (n.s.)
Dalton et al. 2005	Denmark	9743	General population of Denmark	SIR: 0.78 (n.s.)
Goldacre et al. 2005	UK	9649 (number of women unknown)	600 000 individuals with various medical or surgical conditions	RR: 1.17 (n.s.)

IRR, incidence rate ratio (observed/expected number of cases standardized for age and sex); n.s., not statistically significant; s., statistically significant; RR, relative risk; SIR, standardized cancer incidence rate. RR, SIR, IRR < 1 = decreased incidence; RR, SIR, IRR > 1 = increased incidence.

(Osborn *et al.* 2003), hypertension, serious pulmonary disease and prior cardiovascular disease (Curkendall *et al.* 2004).

QTc lengthening: this is a potentially dangerous side-effect of antipsychotic drugs, because it increases the risk of *torsade de pointes* and sudden death

Table 3.26. Population-based studies on the association between schizophrenia and cancer of the corpus uteri

Study	Country	Number of female schizophrenic patients	Control group	Incidence rate for cancer of the corpus uteri in patients with schizophrenia
Mortensen 1989	Denmark	3196	General population of Denmark	IRR: 0.78 (n.s.)
Lawrence et al. 2000	Australia	17 2932 patients with various psychiatric disorders (number of women unknown)	General population of Western Australia	IRR: 0.96 (n.s.)
Lichtermann et al. 2001	Finland	11418	General population of Finland	SIR: 1.75 (s.)
Barak et al. 2005	Israel	3226	General Jewish population of Israel	SIR: 0.24 (n.s.)
Dalton et al. 2005	Denmark	9743	General population of Denmark	SIR: 0.86 (n.s.)
Goldacre et al. 2005	UK	9649 (number of women unknown)	600 000 individuals with various medical or surgical conditions	RR: 1.64 (n.s.)
Grinshpoon et al. 2005	Israel	26 518 (number of women unknown)	General population of Israel	SIR: 1.64 (s.)

IRR, incidence rate ratio (observed/expected number of cases standardized for age and sex); n.s., not statistically significant; RR, relative risk; s., statistically significant; SIR, standardized incidence rate. RR, SIR, IRR < 1 = decreased incidence; RR, SIR, IRR > 1 = increased incidence.

(Reilly *et al.* 2000). Various cut-offs have been suggested, and heart rate adjustment should be made: >440 ms (Meltzer *et al.* 2002), >453 ms (Chong *et al.* 2003), >456 ms (Reilly *et al.* 2000).

Hypertension: defined as a blood pressure ≥140/90 mm Hg or by current use of hypertensive medication (Herold 2002, National Heart, Lung and Blood Institute 2001).

Table 3.27. Population-based studies on the association between schizophrenia and cancer of the ovary

Study	Country	Number of female schizophrenic patients	Control group	Incidence rate for cancer of the ovary in patients with schizophrenia
Mortensen 1989	Denmark	3196	General population of Denmark	IRR: 0.78 (n.s.)
Lawrence et al. 2000	Australia	172 932 patients with various psychiatric disorders (number of women unknown)	General population of Western Australia	IRR: 0.91 (n.s.)
Lichtermann et al. 2001	Finland	11 418	General population of Finland	SIR: 1.22 (n.s.)
Barak et al. 2005	Israel	3226	General Jewish population of Israel	SIR: 0.62 (n.s.)
Dalton et al. 2005	Denmark	9743	General population of Denmark	SIR: 1.14 (n.s.)
Goldacre et al. 2005	UK	9649 (number of women unknown)	600 000 individuals with various medical or surgical conditions	RR: 1.05 (n.s.)

IRR, incidence rate ratio (observed/expected number of cases standardized for age and sex); n.s., not statistically significant; RR, relative risk; SIR, standardized incidence rate. RR, SIR, IRR < 1 = decreased incidence; RR, SIR, IRR > 1 = increased incidence.

Hypotension: defined as a systolic blood pressure 100 mm Hg (systolic) (Herold 2002).

Postural hypotension: has been defined as a drop in excess of 20 mm Hg in systolic blood pressure and of 10 mm Hg in diastolic blood pressure after standing up from a lying position (Silver *et al.* 1990).

Sudden cardiac death: a sudden pulseless condition (arrest) that proved fatal (within 48 hours) and was consistent with ventricular tachyarrhythmia occurring in the absence of a known non-cardiac condition as the proximate cause of the death (Siscovick *et al.* 1994).

It is a common notion of psychiatric textbooks that the risk of cardiovascular problems is increased in patients with schizophrenia. Most of the epidemiological evidence stems from mortality studies which have consistently shown that people with schizophrenia die more frequently from cardiovascular diseases and suffer sudden death than control populations (Allebeck 1989, Brown *et al.* 2000, Goldman 1999, Newman and Bland 1991). Studies on cardiovascular *comorbidity* – which are the focus of our review – were more scarce than expected, given the importance of the problem. However, 21 high-quality population-based studies were identified. Table 3.28 summarizes those studies that used a control group as a minimum criterion. Studies that solely measured cardiovascular mortality rather than cardiovascular comorbidity were excluded, because the former have been well summarized in earlier reviews (e.g. Brown *et al.* 2000, Harris and Barraclough 1998). In addition, studies that examined the cardiac effects of antipsychotic medications were included only if they used a control group of non-schizophrenic subjects.

Overall, the studies confirm that people with schizophrenia have higher rates of cardiovascular problems than normal controls. However, when specific cardiovascular problems are considered, the picture becomes more heterogeneous. For example, four studies showed that hypertension is less frequent in patients with schizophrenia (Schwalb 1975, Schwalb *et al.* 1976, Silver *et al.* 1990, Steinert *et al.* 1996) compared to normal controls. Dixon *et al.* (1999) reported high frequencies of hypertension, but they had no normal control group, only control groups with other psychiatric disorders. Low blood pressure in people with schizophrenia can probably be explained by the effects of some antipsychotic drugs on alpha and muscarinergic receptors.

The main factors explaining the increased frequency of cardiovascular problems are likely to be linked to the accumulation of a number of the risk factors summarized above: high rates of smoking, weight gain, diabetes, dyslipidemia and lack of exercise are all associated with schizophrenia (de Leon and Diaz 2005, Dixon *et al.* 2000, Marder *et al.* 2004, National Institutes of Health 2004, Ryan *et al.* (2003)). In addition, part of the morbidity may be caused by the well-known cardiac effects of antipsychotic drugs. A detailed review of medication side-effects would go beyond the scope of this review, but some antipsychotics cause QTc prolongation, other arrhythmias and thrombosis, have alpha-adrenergic and muscarinergic effects; also cases of myocarditis during clozapine use have been reported. Finally, Lawrence *et al.* (2003) argued that stigma may be an important factor in increased cardiac morbidity and mortality, because in their study revascularization procedures were offered much more seldom to patients with schizophrenia than to normal controls. In a similar vein Davidson (2002) pointed out that system-related barriers (e.g. lack of insurance coverage, lack of access to healthcare, stigmatization, lack of integration of medical and mental health systems) and patient-related barriers (poverty, non-compliance,

Table 3.28. Studies on the risk of cardiovascular diseases in patients with schizophrenia

Study	Country	Study period	Research question	Number of patients with schizophrenia (S) and control group (C)	Number of cardiovascular events	Data source on schizophrenia and cardiovascular diseases	Conclusions
Schwalb 1975	Germany	2 years	Prevalence of coronary heart disease in hospitalized psychiatric patients (between 40–69 years, mean hospitalization: 15.7 years) compared with the results of some epidemiological studies in average populations	Total psychiatric patients: 1726 S: 809 C: general population	Constant hypertension: Men 40–49 years: 10.7% vs. 18.8% Men 50–49 years: 16.3% vs. 25% Women 29.1% vs. 42.8% Pathologic ECG: Men 40–49 years: 0.5% vs. 17.6% Men 50–59 years: 12.7% vs. 22.7%	Patients from eight different hospitals in Germany Control data: Blackburn *et al.* 1960, Blohmke *et al.* 1970	Lower prevalence of hypertension and pathologic ECG in psychiatric patients compared to results from studies on the German general population

Reference	Country	Aim	Sample	Results	Notes	Conclusion
Lovett Doust 1980	Canada	Prevalence of sinus tachycardia and abnormal cardiac rate in outpatients with schizophrenia compared to healthy controls	S: 138, 57 without psychotropic drugs, 81 with psychotropic drugs C: 139	Mean sinus rhythm heart rate in beats/min: S: without psychotropic drugs: 84, with psychotropic drugs: 88.7 C: 73.9 ECG changes: S: 42%	not available	Higher sinus rhythm heart rates in both treated and untreated patients with schizophrenia compared to control subjects; the rate tended to increase with treatment
Silver et al. 1990	Israel	Prevalence of postural hypotension in schizophrenic patients on stable antipsychotic treatment (minimum hospitalization: 2 years, median hospitalization: 10 years) compared with unmedicated healthy controls	S: 200 C: 25	Mean blood pressure (RRBP) at rest (mm Hg): 119.1/64.9 vs. 125.8/78.2 Mean RRBP at 1 min: 91.0/58.8 vs. 129.4/88.6 Mean RRBP at 3 min: 109.1/62.6 vs. 126.8/88.0 Postural hypotension[a]: S: at 1 min: 77%, at 3 min: 16.8% C: 0%	Hospital records of consenting chronic schizophrenic patients from the Flugelman (Mazra) Psychiatric Hospital; the control group was recruited from the hospital staff	Significantly lower resting blood pressure among and significantly higher prevalence of postural hypotension in schizophrenic patients compared to controls

95

Table 3.28. (*cont.*)

Study	Country	Study period	Research question	Number of patients with schizophrenia (S) and control group (C)	Number of cardiovascular events	Data source on schizophrenia and cardiovascular diseases	Conclusions
Steinert *et al.* 1996	Germany	3 years	Cardiovascular morbidity in long-term hospitalized patients with schizophrenia (mean age 62.6 years, mean duration of hospitalization 28.6 years) compared to corresponding data from the German population	S: 90 (43 men/47 women) C: General population of Germany	RRBP systolic (men/women in mm Hg): S: 126.8/127.2 C: 139.2/136.0 RRBP diastolic (men/women in mm Hg): S: 79.3/78.2 C: 85.4/82.0	Hospital records of all inpatients of the Psychiatric Hospital of Weissenau who were hospitalized for at least 5 years and who were at least 40 years old. General population data: Bundesgesundheitsministerium der BRD 1991	Systolic and diastolic blood pressure was lower in schizophrenic subjects than in the corresponding age of the general population

Study	Country	Aim	Sample	Results	Conclusion
Warner et al. 1996	UK	Prevalence of electrocardiographic changes in psychiatric inpatients (90% with schizophrenia, 3% bipolar disorders, 4% depression and 3% undetermined, dementia excluded) aged under 75 (mean age 51 years) receiving neuroleptic medication compared to unmedicated controls (mean age 47 years)	Patients with neuroleptic treatment: 111 C: 42	Mean heart rate: Medicated group: 83 C: 72 (s.) Mean QTc (ms): Medicated group: 404.3 C: 387.7 (s.) Mean QRS (ms): Medicated group: 96.5 C: 92.2 (n.s.) Mean PR interval: Medicated group: 151.2 C: 151.8 (n.s.)	Controls from the hospital staff	High prevalence of QTc prolongation in psychiatric patients. QTc interval prolongation was more likely in patients on doses above 2000 mg chlorpromazine equivalents daily. No significant difference between PR and QRS intervals between psychiatric patients and control group
Dixon et al. 1999	USA	Prevalence of medical comorbidities in in- and outpatients with schizophrenia (mean age 43 years) with antipsychotic treatment compared with two cohorts from the general population.	S: 719 C: general population (NHIS 1994) C1: 18–44 years C2: 45–64 years	Hypertension: lifetime: 34.1%, current: 19.3% C1: 5.1% C2: 22.2% Heart problems: lifetime: 15.6%, current: 11.6% C1: 3.8% C2: 13.6%	Patient Outcomes Research Team Survey in two states, one in the South and the other in the Midwest, face-to-face interviews, National Health Interview Survey 1994	Overall, the current rates of both hypertension and heart disease of persons with schizophrenia resemble those of the older cohort of the general population

Table 3.28. (*cont.*)

Study	Country	Study period	Research question	Number of patients with schizophrenia (S) and control group (C)	Number of cardiovascular events	Data source on schizophrenia and cardiovascular diseases	Conclusions
Munck-Jorgensen *et al.* 2000	Denmark		Analysis of RateR for schizophrenic patients' admissions to somatic departments in Denmark; comparison with age- and sex-matched controls	S: 20 000 C: 20 0000	Severe heart failure: RateR: 4.15 Atherosclerotic disease of the brain vessels: RateR: 0.35	Danish Psychiatric Central Register, Danish Central Person Register, Danish National Patient Register	Higher RateR for severe heart failure and decreased RateR for atherosclerotic disease of the brain vessels. It seems that individuals with schizophrenia are rarely treated for their physical illness in its early, less severe phases, but more likely in its acute phases when the disease is severe, life-threatening or painful

Author	Country	Years	Aim	Sample	Results	Setting	Conclusions
Reilly et al. 2000	UK	1994–6	Point prevalence of QTc lengthening in psychiatric patients and the effect of various psychotropic drugs compared with healthy reference individuals	Total psychiatric patients: 495 S: 217 C: 101	QTc lengthening in total psychiatric patients: 8% No numbers for schizophrenics and control group given	Participants were patients of all mental health facilities in six districts in north-east England who gave their written consent; the healthy comparison group was recruited from the hospital staff	Age over 65 years, use of tricyclic antidepressants, thioridazine, and droperidol and high-dose antipsychotic treatment were robust predictors of QTc lengthening; lithium was associated with abnormal QT dispersion or T-wave abnormalities
Cohen et al. 2001	Israel		Association of heart rate variability and risk for sudden death in patients with schizophrenia on long-term psychotropic medication compared to age, gender, smoking and time of ray of ECG recordings-matched healthy, unmedicated controls	S: 56 clozapine: 21 haloperidol: 18 olanzapine: 17 C: 53	Mean heart rate: S: clozapine: 107 (s.) S: haloperidol: 85.8 (s.) S: olanzapine: 89.05 (s.) C: 62 (s.) Mean QTc (ms): S: clozapine: 502.9 (s.) S: haloperidol: 517.8 (s.) S: olanzapine: 504.6 (s.) C: 370 (s.)	In- and outpatient treatment programmes at the Beer-Sheva Mental Health Centre	Significantly higher heart rate in patients with schizophrenia on clozapine, haloperidol and olanzapine and prolonged QTc intervals in patients with any neuroleptic treatment compared to healthy controls

Table 3.28. (cont.)

Study	Country	Study period	Research question	Number of patients with schizophrenia (S) and control group (C)	Number of cardiovascular events	Data source on schizophrenia and cardiovascular diseases	Conclusions
Davidson et al. 2001	Australia		Cross-sectional survey of cardiovascular risk factors (smoking, alcohol consumption, overweight and obesity, lack of exercise, hypertension, salt intake, hypercholesterolaemia) among outpatients with mental illness between 18 and 65 years compared with a community sample from the general population	Chronic psychiatric patients (79% with psychotic disorder) (PS): 234 C: general population	Smoking: PS: 61.9% C: 23.7% (s.) Alcohol: moderate[b]: PS: 25.2% C: 52.3% (s.) harmful[c]: PS: 11.5% C: 3.1% (s.) BMI: overweight: PS: 27.8% C: 22.7% (s.) obese: PS: 39.7% C: 7.8% (s.) Exercise (no exercise): PS: 29.1% C: 28.1% (n.s.)	Patients from a community mental health clinic in the North-western Health Care Network in Melbourne	Higher prevalence of smoking, overweight and obesity, lack of moderate exercise, harmful levels of alcohol consumption and salt intake in psychiatric outpatients compared with the general population; no differences were found on hypertension

Study	Country	Years	Aim	Number of participants	Results	Data source	Conclusion
Ray et al. 2001	USA	1989–93	Prevalence of sudden cardiac death in antipsychotic users between 15 and 84 years compared to persons without any antipsychotic medication	Number of total psychiatric patients: 481 744 Follow-up (in person-years): total: 1 282 996 medication in the past year only: 37 881 current low-dose antipsychotic use (= 100 mg): 31 864 current moderate-dose antipsychotic use (>100 mg): 26 749 C (no medication): 1 186 501	Multivariate rate ratio of sudden cardiac death: medication in the past year only: 1.20 (n.s.) current use (= 100mg): 1.30 (n.s.) current use (>100mg): 2.39, (s.) C: 1 (referent)	Tennessee Medicaid enrolees, Medicaid pharmacy files, Tennessee death certificates	Increased risk of sudden cardiac death in moderate-dose antipsychotic users

Table 3.28. (*cont.*)

Study	Country	Study period	Research question	Number of patients with schizophrenia (S) and control group (C)	Number of cardiovascular events	Data source on schizophrenia and cardiovascular diseases	Conclusions
Hennessy *et al.* 2002	USA	1993–6	Prevalence of cardiac arrest and ventricular arrhythmia in outpatients with antipsychotic treated schizophrenia compared with a control group with glaucoma and another control group with psoriasis	S: 8330 (clozapine), 41 295 (haloperidol), 22 057 (risperidone), 23 950 (thioridazine) C: 7541 (psoriasis drug), 21 545 (glaucoma drug)	Rate per 1000 person years: Cardiac arrest and ventricular arrhythmia: S: clozapine: 2.2 (s.) S: haloperidol: 4.2 (s.) S: risperidone: 5.0 (s.) S: thioridazine: 3.8 (s.) C: psoriasis drug: 1.8 (s.) glaucoma drug: 3.4 (s.)	3 US Medicaid programmes	Higher rates of cardiac arrest and ventricular arrhythmia in patients with schizophrenia than in controls. Thioridazine was not worse than haloperidol. However, thioridazine may have a higher risk at high doses

| Chong et al. 2003 | Singapore | Prevalence of prolonged QTc intervals in patients with schizophrenia with typical antipsychotic medication (mean age 51.3 years) compared with healthy controls (mean age 51.6 years) | S: 163 C: 100 | Adjusted OR: Prolonged QTc (<456 ms): S: chlorpromazine: 13.5 (s.) S: trifluoperazine: 0.5 (n.s.) S: flupenthixol decanoate: 34.1 (s.) S: zuclopenthixol decanoate: 7.0 (n.s.) S: Haloperidol: 3.9 (n.s.) S: Thioridazine: 13.9 (n.s.) S: Fluphenazine decanoate: 13.7 (s.) S: Lithium: 0.5 (n.s.) S: Carbamazepine: 0.4, n.s. C: Prolonged QTc (>453 ms): 6.7% | Patients from the Woodbridge Hospital, the only state mental institute in Singapore; controls from the hospital staff | Significant predictors for QTc lengthening were use of chlorpromazine, flupenthixol decanoate, and fluphenazine decanoate |

Table 3.28. (*cont.*)

Study	Country	Study period	Research question	Number of patients with schizophrenia (S) and control group (C)	Number of cardiovascular events	Data source on schizophrenia and cardiovascular diseases	Conclusions
Lawrence et al. 2003	Australia	1980–98	Population-based record linkage study to investigate the association between mental illness and rates of revascularization procedures in psychiatric patients compared to the general population	Psychiatric patients: 210 129 S: 9721 C: 1 831 399 (general population)	Admission RateR for IHD: AMI: men: 0.96 (n.s.), women: 0.93 (s.) Other acute and subacute IHD: men: 1.34 (s.), women: 1.47 (s.) AP: men: 1.10 (s.), women: 1.25 (s.) Coronary atherosclerosis: men: 0.91 (s.), women: 1.16 (s.) Other IHD: men: 1.09 (n.s.), women: 1.30 (s.)	Western Australian Health Service Linked Database	Little difference in hospital admission rates for IHD between psychiatric patients and the general community, but much lower rates of revascularization procedures with psychiatric patients, particularly in people with psychoses

Study	Country	Aim	Sample	Results	Setting	Conclusion
				Total (all disorders): men: 0.99 (n.s.), women: 1.10 (s.), S: men: 0.59 (s.), women: 0.60 (s.). Revascularization procedure rate ratio: S: men: 0.31 (s.), women: 0.34(s.). C: removal of coronary artery obstruction: men 0.85 (s.), women: 0.98 (n.s.) C: coronary artery bypass graft or arterial implant: men 0.75 (s.), women: 0.90 (n.s.)		
Cohn *et al.* 2004	Canada	Prevalence of coronary heart disease risk factors in patients with chronic schizophrenia or schizoaffective disorder compared with rates in the US general population	S: 240 C1: 7020 C2: US general population	Framingham 10-year risk of MI: Men: S: 8.9%, C1: 6.3% (s.). Women: S: 2.6%, C1: 2.0% Metabolic syndrome: Men: S: 42.6%, C2: 24% Women S: 48.5%, C2: 23%	In- and outpatients from the Schizophrenia Program at the Centre for Addiction and Mental Health in Toronto, Ontario. Control group 1: from the Canadian Heart Health Survey; control group 2: US adult population	Greater Framingham 10-year risk of MI in the male patients, but not in females compared with the Canadian reference group. Prevalence rates of metabolic syndrome in patients were approximately two times rates in the US adult population

Table 3.33. Leukaemia

Study	Country	Number of schizophrenic patients	Control group	Incidence rate for leukaemia in patients with schizophrenia
Mortensen 1989	Denmark	6152: men: 2956, women: 3196	General population of Denmark	IRR: men: 1.02 (n.s.), women: 0.65 (n.s.)
Lawrence et al. 2000	Australia	172 932 patients with various psychiatric disorders (number of men and women unknown)	General population of Western Australia	RR: men: 0.86 (n.s.), women: 0.97 (n.s.)
Dalton et al. 2005	Denmark	22 766: men: 13 023, women: 9743	General population of Denmark	SIR: men : 0.99 (n.s.), women: 0.74 (n.s.)
Goldacre et al. 2005	UK	9649	600 000 hospital patients in the Oxford Health Region	RR: 0.94 (n.s.)

IRR, incidence rate ratio (observed/expected number of cases standardized for age and sex); n.s., not statistically significant; RR, relative risk; SIR, standardized incidence rate. RR, SIR, IRR < 1 = decreased incidence; RR, SIR, IRR > 1 = increased incidence.

from the population-based incidence studies on cancer in the section on Neoplasms (section 3.4). The data are very heterogeneous, with no studies showing statistically significant results. This research suffers from limited statistical power and its results are inconclusive.

3.16. Congenital, hereditary and neonatal diseases and abnormalities

The MEDLINE search on *Congenital, Hereditary and Neonatal Diseases and Abnormalities* yielded 1042 hits. Ten reports were ordered, but only one relevant report was included. One report was added by cross-referencing. This category overlapped with a number of other topics so that many studies were transferred to other chapters.

3.16.1. Klinefelter's syndrome

Negulici and Christodorescu (1967) described a case with co-occurring Kline-felter's syndrome and schizophrenia. They also reviewed the literature and found that people with Klinefelter's syndrome often have manifestations of schizophrenic symptoms.

3.16.2. Neurological abnormalities

Schubert and McNeil (2004) compared neurological abnormalities in 75 young adult offspring of mothers having psychotic disorders with 91 offspring of mothers having no history of psychosis. They found high levels of neurological abnormalities in a substantial proportion of the offspring of mothers with schizophrenia. They suggested that familial risk for schizophrenia may be associated with neurodevelopmental disturbances.

3.17. Skin and connective tissue diseases

The MEDLINE search on *Skin and Connective Tissue Diseases* yielded 379 hits, of which 35 reports were ordered. From these, 28 reports were included and 22 reports were added by cross-referencing.

3.17.1. Allergic skin reactions

Sugerman *et al.* (1982) found increased immunoglobulin E (IgE) antibodies – a marker of allergy – in depression and schizophrenia. Rybakowski *et al.* (1992) investigated the prevalence of allergic skin reactions by intradermal tests. They studied 60 psychiatric patients (30 with a diagnosis of schizophrenia) and found a prevalence of hypersensitivity of 27% in patients with schizophrenia and 40% in patients with affective disorders.

3.17.2. Hyperpigmentation of the skin

Robins (1972) investigated the effects of prolonged treatment with phenothiazines on the skin melanin concentration in 182 phenothiazine-treated chronic schizophrenics, 182 matched drug-treated (phenytoin and/or phenothiazines) control patients (epileptics, patients with mental subnormality, alcoholic psychosis and other organic psycho-syndromes) and 163 normal subjects. The schizophrenic patients had significantly higher skin melanin concentrations than the normal controls, but they did not differ in melanin content from the drug-treated controls. Robins concluded that melanosis is a non-specific response to the phenothiazines and not caused by schizophrenia itself.

Ban *et al.* (1985) reviewed studies on the occurrence of phenothiazine-induced skin pigmentation. Skin pigmentation occurred in 1.0% to 2.9% in schizophrenic patients, with a greater prevalence in females and in patients treated with chlorpromazine. Ban *et al.* (1985) surveyed 768 chronic hospitalized schizophrenic patients in the framework of a multi-national collaborative study and found a prevalence rate of 1.7%. No definitive relationships between sex, diagnosis, drugs, dosage of medication and skin pigmentation were found.

In summary, all this literature on hyperpigmentation is related to the effects of some antipsychotic drugs, but no evidence going beyond this side-effect is available.

3.17.3. Lupus erythematodes

Medication-induced lupus erythematodes had already been described in 1951 by Gold (cited by Gallien *et al.* 1975; no reference available). Gallien *et al.* (1975) investigated 600 psychiatric inpatients treated with phenothiazines and found positive reactions of lupus-associated antinuclear bodies in 23.1%. They speculated that the antinuclear bodies were caused by antipsychotic treatment and that the titres depended on dosage and duration of exposure.

3.17.4. Tuberous sclerosis

Herkert *et al.* (1972) reported cases of the coincidence of tuberous sclerosis and schizophrenia. Tuberous sclerosis is characterized by proliferative lesions in the brain, the retina, the skin, many visceral organs and the bones. The case reports described only psychotic features in patients with tuberous sclerosis and not the frequency of occurrence of tuberous sclerosis in patients with schizophrenia.

3.17.5. Pellagra

Hoffer (1970) compared pellagra and schizophrenia. Pellagra is caused by a dietary deficiency of vitamin B_3 (nicotinic acid and/or nicotinamide (NAD)) and can cause psychotic symptoms. Other symptoms are dermatitis, dementia and diarrhoea. Hoffer (1970) suggested that schizophrenia might also be caused by a deficiency of NAD, because the synthesis of NAD is disturbed. He believed that if the vitamin B_3 intake is adequate, pellagra and schizophrenia remain latent.

Another report, by Dickerson and Wiryanti (1978), investigated mental changes in pellagra. They suggested that interrelationships of tryptophan, nicotinic acid and amino acid imbalance might be involved in brain serotonin metabolism in the psychiatric disturbances of pellagra, depression and possibly also schizophrenia.

Table 3.34. Skin cancer

Study	Country	Number of schizophrenic patients	Control group	Incidence rate for skin cancer in patients with schizophrenia
Mortensen 1994	Denmark	9156: men: 5658, women: 3498	General population of Denmark	SIR: men: 0.24 (s.), women: 0.87 (n.s.)
Barak et al. 2005	Israel	3226	General Jewish population of Israel	SIR: 0.13 (s.)
Dalton et al. 2005	Denmark	22 766: men: 13 023, women: 9743	General population of Denmark	SIR: men: 0.77 (s.), women: 0.81 (n.s.)
Goldacre et al. 2005	UK	9649	600 000 hospital patients in the Oxford Health Region	RR: 0.56 (s.)

n.s., not statistically significant; RR, relative risk; s., statistically significant; SIR, standardized incidence rate. RR, SIR < 1 = decreased incidence; RR, SIR > 1 = increased incidence.

3.17.6.   Skin cancer and malignant melanoma

Tables 3.34 and 3.35 provide a summary of the results on the frequency of skin cancer and malignant melanoma and were derived from the section on neoplasms (section 3.4). The studies reviewed there were analysed as to results on forms of skin cancer. There was a risk reduction for skin cancer and malignant melanoma. A possible hypothetical explanation could be that schizophrenic patients are less exposed to risk factors for these cancers, e.g. sunbathing (Osterlind 1990).

3.17.7.   Rheumatoid arthritis

There were 18 epidemiological studies on the association between schizophrenia and rheumatoid arthritis (RA).

Nissen and Spencer (1936) noticed a negative association between schizophrenia and RA as early as 1936. Numerous studies followed theirs, the last one identified having been published in 2006. Important characteristics of these trials are summarized in Table 3.36. As many as 15 of 18 studies investigating several tens of thousands of inpatients found a negative association between schizophrenia and RA. Two small studies (Krakowski et al. 1983, Ramsay et al. 1982), which together involved only 665 schizophrenia patients, found a

Table 3.35. Malignant melanoma

Study	Country	Number of schizophrenic patients	Control group	Incidence rate for malignant melanoma in patients with schizophrenia
Mortensen 1989	Denmark	6152: men: 2956, women: 3196	General population of Denmark	IRR: men: 1.17 (n.s.), women: 1.12 (n.s.)
Mortensen 1994	Denmark	9156: men: 5658, women: 3498	General population of Denmark	SIR: men: 0.00 (s.), women: 0.26 (n.s.)
Dalton *et al.* 2005	Denmark	22 766: men: 13 023, women: 9743	General population of Denmark	SIR: men: 0.59 (n.s.), women: 0.69 (n.s.)
Goldacre *et al.* 2005	UK	9649	600 000 hospital patients in the Oxford Health Region	RR: 0.20 (s.)
Grinshpoon *et al.* 2005	Israel	26 518 (number of men and women not given)	General population of Israel	SIR: men: 0.86 (n.s.), women: 0.47 (s.)

IRR, incidence rate ratio (observed/expected number of cases standardized for age and sex); n.s., not statistically significant; RR, relative risk; s., statistically significant; SIR, standardized incidence rate. RR, SIR, IRR < 1 = decreased incidence; RR, SIR, IRR > 1 = increased incidence.

frequency of RA similar to that in the general population. One population-based study, by Lauerma *et al.* (1998), also failed to support the negative association between schizophrenia and RA. The authors examined a Finnish birth cohort and found numerically higher incidence rates of RA in the schizophrenic cohort members (1.3%) compared to members without psychiatric diagnosis (0.46%). Oken and Schulzer 1999 summarized the nine studies with the most complete data in a meta-analysis and found that schizophrenia patients had a relative risk for polyarthritis of 29% compared to *other psychiatric patients*. They argued that compared to the *general population* – in which the risk has been reported to be 1% (Spector 1990) – the relative risk might be even much lower.

A long list of hypotheses has been proposed to explain the rarity of cases with RA in schizophrenia. The main hypotheses are summarized in Table 3.37 and an excellent discussion has been provided by Torrey and Yolken (2001).

However, especially the early studies have also been criticized for a number of methodological problems (for review see e.g. Eaton *et al.* 1992, Mors *et al.* 1999, Oken and Schulzer 1999).

Many studies had no control group or if they did, the schizophrenia group was compared with a sample of patients with other psychiatric diagnoses rather than with normal controls.

Failure to consider age and gender in a study may lead to bias. The prevalence of RA is higher in females while a recent meta-analysis suggested that the prevalence of schizophrenia might be slightly higher in men (Aleman *et al.* 2003). Both diseases also differ in typical age of onset (Eaton *et al.* 1992).

The early studies did not use appropriate diagnostic criteria and many studies used only medical records or unspecific screening to identify cases. Cases of RA might have been overlooked by such a procedure, leading to erroneously low comorbidity rates. Considering the fact that diagnostic criteria for schizophrenia suggested by the International Classification of Diseases (ICD-10) or the Diagnostic and Statistical Manual of Mental Disorders (DSM-IV) have been narrowed compared to early criteria, it is difficult to compare the old studies with the more recent ones.

Further problems are the low number of patients included in a number of reports and the fact that very few studies were population based. Furthermore, almost all studies were carried out on hospitalized patients. Although this had the advantage that the more severely ill patients were considered so that the researchers could be clearer about their diagnoses, low prevalences of RA have also been found in other institutionalized populations such as prisoners (Rothermich and Philips 1963). Environmental factors could thus contribute to the low comorbidity.

Antipsychotic medication was not considered as a confounding or explanatory factor in most studies. It has been argued that antipsychotic drugs may have analgesic effects and that they may suppress the immune system. However, a number of the studies summarized in Table 3.36 were published in the pre-neuroleptic era.

Mors *et al.* (1999) stressed that the most important confounder may be under-reporting of RA by patients with schizophrenia. In an elegant population-based study they applied both a retrospective case-control design and a prospective follow-up study. Both studies confirmed the decreased rates of RA in schizophrenia. However, they found that the rates of diseases such as osteoarthritis and even unspecific back pain in schizophrenia were also decreased, confirming the results of e.g. Mohamed *et al.* (1982). Since the latter disorders are not known to be associated with genetic factors, the authors argue that the simplest explanation for the association is still a reduced tendency to report musculoskeletal pain by patients with schizophrenia rather than any aetiological hypothesis. This behaviour may be due to neglect because of the psychosis, a greater pain

Table 3.36. Schizophrenia and rheumatoid arthritis (RA)

Study	Country	Research question	Number of patients with schizophrenia (S), psychiatric patients in general (P), control group (C)	Number of patients with RA	Data sources on schizophrenia and RA, diagnostic criteria	Result
Nissen and Spencer 1936	Not reported	Prevalence of arthritis of all types in a psychiatric hospital	P: 2200 inpatients with various mental disorders	P: 0	Not reported	No case of RA observed
Gregg 1939	USA (Massachusetts)	Information by nine Massachusetts hospital superintendents about the prevalence of RA in inpatients with psychosis	P: 10 993 psychotic inpatients, age > 40 years C: general population of Massachusetts	P: 18 C: No data	Questionnaire sent to hospital	Frequency of 0.16% in patients with a psychiatric diagnosis other than schizophrenia, no data given for schizophrenia
Ross et al. 1950	Canada (Quebec)	Prevalence of RA in inpatients with schizophrenia and in non-schizophrenic psychiatric inpatients	S: 800 inpatients P: 808 inpatients with other psychiatric diagnoses	S: 0 P: 4	Medical records history, physical and radiological examinations	No case of RA in patients with schizophrenia, frequency of RA in patients with other psychiatric diagnosis 0.49%
Trevathan and Tatum 1954	USA (Alabama)	Prevalence of RA in discharge records from a neuropsychiatric hospital	P: 9000 inpatients	P: 1	Discharge diagnosis	No case of RA in patients with schizophrenia, frequency of RA in patients with other psychiatric diagnosis 0.011%

Study	Country	Aim	Sample	n with RA	Methods	Results
Pilkington 1956	UK	Prevalence of RA in female inpatients with various psychiatric diagnoses	S: 130 female inpatients, age >40 P: 188 female inpatients with other psychiatric diagnoses, age >40	S: 1 P: 5	History, physical, radiological and ESR ARA criteria	Schizophrenia patients: 0.77%, patients with other psychiatric diagnosis: 2.7%
Ehrentheil 1957	USA (Massachusetts)	Prevalence of RA in inpatients of a neuropsychiatric hospital	P: 4500 inpatients with various psychiatric diagnoses	P: 1	Medical records	Frequency of 0.22% in patients with various psychiatric diagnoses
Rothermich and Philips 1963	USA (Ohio)	Prevalence of RA in psychiatric inpatients	P1: 16000 psychotic inpatients, P2: 4494 non-psychotic inpatients	P1: 13 P2: 17	Unspecified screening, physical, radiological and serological exams; ARA criteria	Frequency of 0.08% in psychotic patients and 0.38% in non-psychotic inpatients
Mellsop et al. 1974	Australia	Investigation about the prevalence of RA in middle-aged women (mean age 53.1 years) with a substantiated diagnosis of schizophrenia selected from various psychiatric hospitals	S: 301 female inpatients. No control group	S: 0	Victorian Psychiatric Hospitals, Australia, comparison with large population studies	Significant difference ($p < 0.001$) between the observed vs. the expected prevalence (nil vs. 23)

Table 3.36. (*cont.*)

Study	Country	Research question	Number of patients with schizophrenia (S), psychiatric patients in general (P), control group (C)	Number of patients with RA	Data sources on schizophrenia and RA, diagnostic criteria	Result
Osterberg 1978	Sweden	In the main analysis the discharge diagnoses of all Swedish patients with schizophrenia were compared with those of patients with other psychiatric diagnoses	S: 40 426 inpatients P: 142 406 inpatients with other psychiatric disorders	S: 19 P: 149	Discharge diagnoses available to the Swedish National Social Welfare Board	Low frequency of RA in schizophrenic patients of 0.047% compared to 0.11% in other psychiatric patients. However, even the RA rate of other psychiatric patients was low
Baldwin 1979	UK	Prevalence of RA in psychiatric patients of two counties in England from an 8-year period	S: 2314 inpatients P: 5404 inpatients with other psychiatric diagnoses	S: 2 P: 23	Oxford Record Linkage Study, ICD-8 revision criteria	Schizophrenia patients: 0.09%, patients with other psychiatric diagnosis: 0.43%
Mohamed et al. 1982	Canada	Comparison of the frequency of RA and other connective tissue diseases in schizophrenic patients (mean age 49.5 years) versus age-matched (mean age 52.2 years) inpatients with other psychiatric conditions	S: 111 P: 51	S: 0 P: 3	Medical records of London Psychiatric Hospital, Ontario	No case of RA in the schizophrenia group, but three in the control group

Study	Country	Description	Sample		Method	Results
Ramsay et al. 1982	Canada, USA	Epidemiological study about the relationship between schizophrenia and certain 'psychosomatic' illnesses (peptic ulcer, bronchial asthma, neurodermatitis and RA); 354 patients, age range 20–70 years, from chronic and general hospitals with the diagnosis of schizophrenia	S: 354: chronic hospital: 198, general hospital: 156. No control group	S: 12	Clinical interview, medical, psychiatric and psychoso-matic history, confirmation of the patient's psychiatrist, laboratory and radiological tests	RA had the lowest overall prevalence (3.4%, s.) in patients with schizophrenia, the male–female differences (1.8% vs. 6.1%) were not statistically significant. Each of the four disorders was more highly represented in the general hospital as compared to the chronic hospital population
Krakowski et al. 1983	Poland	Prevalence of RA in a group of Polish schizophrenia patients	S: 311, ages 20–70 No control group	S: 8	History, unspecified laboratory tests, radiological examination	Frequency of 2.6% in schizophrenic patients

Table 3.36. (*cont.*)

Study	Country	Research question	Number of patients with schizophrenia (S), psychiatric patients in general (P), control group (C)	Number of patients with RA	Data sources on schizophrenia and RA, diagnostic criteria	Result
Allebeck *et al.* 1985	Sweden	Follow-up study about the incidence of hospital care with the diagnosis RA among patients with schizophrenia compared with that among patients with ther psychiatric diagnosis and non-psychiatric patients. Calculation of SMR (observed and expected incidence). Period of observation: 1971–81	S: 1190 inpatients, P1: 621 affective psychosis P2: 3978 neurosis C: 10 152 medical, non-psychiatric inpatients	S: 2 P1: 2 P2: 17 C: 71	Stockholm county medical information system; population register of Sweden; inpatient register of Stockholm County with the diagnosis of schizophrenia and with any other psychiatric diagnosis (control group); cause-of-death register	Incidence of RA was around half the expected incidence in schizophrenic patients: ratio, males and females combined = 0.17 vs. 0.43 (reference group); SMR = 0.4 (n.s.)

Author	Country	Aim/Methods	Sample	Source	Results
Lauerma et al. 1998	Finland	Examination of the incidence of schizophrenia and RA among a birth cohort ($n = 11\,017$) born in 1966	S: 76 P: 438 C: 10 503 without any psychiatric diagnosis	Finnish Hospital Discharge Register, DSM – III – R criteria	Incidence of RA in schizophrenic patients: 1.3%; first control group: 0.29%, second control group: 0.46%
Mors et al. 1999	Denmark	Population-based case control (1) and follow-up study (2) about the association between schizophrenia and RA before or after the first ever admission for schizophrenia; 20 495 schizophrenics compared with 204 912 persons matched on age and gender from the general population; estimation of odds ratio and relative risks by Mantel–Haenszel estimator and Poisson regression. Period of observation: 1978–93	S: 20 495 C: 204 912 (general population) (1) Case-control study: S: 11 C: 2502 (2) Follow-up study: S: 22 C: no data available	Danish Psychiatric Case Register; National Patient Register: control group Danish Central Person Register	(1) Case-control study: negative association between RA and schizophrenia for females (OR 0.46, s.) and the two sexes combined (OR 0.44, s.). For males reduced risk, but not statistically significant (OR = 0.41, n.s.) (2) Follow-up study: Negative association between schizophrenia and the occurrence of RA: men: OR 0.22(s.), women: OR 0.30 (s.), both sexes combined: OR 0.28 (s.)

Table 3.36. (*cont.*)

Study	Country	Research question	Number of patients with schizophrenia (S), psychiatric patients in general (P), control group (C)	Number of patients with RA	Data sources on schizophrenia and RA, diagnostic criteria	Result
Oken and Schulzer 1999	USA (New York)	Prevalence of RA in schizophrenia patients; comparison with 661 non-schizophrenia inpatients	S: 1323 P: 661	S: 1 P: 2	Patients in Pilgrim State Psychiatric Center, West Brentwood, NY on 24 July 1993, DSM-III-R criteria, ARA diagnostic criteria	RA comorbidity frequency of 0.076%, control group: 0.30%

Oken and Schulzer 1999	Canada	Prevalence of RA in schizophrenia patients adjusted for deaths and readmissions (age >18) in Canada in comparison to psychiatric patients without the diagnosis of schizophrenia. Period of observation: 1984–88	S: 27 630 inpatients P: 202 342	S: 30 P: 900	Canadian hospital separation statistics, ICD-9 diagnostic criteria	RA frequency in schizophrenia patients: 0.11% (s.), in other psychiatric patients: 0.44% (s.)
Eaton et al. 2006	Denmark	Prevalence of RA in patients with schizophrenia. Period of observation: 1981–98	S: 7704 C: 192 590	Seropositive RA: S: 10 C: 234 Seronegative RA: S: 5 C: 102	Danish Psychiatric Register, Danish National Patient Register	Seropositive RA prevalence (per 1000) in schizophrenia patients: 0.13, control group: 0.12. Other RA prevalence: 0.06 vs. 0.05.

ARA, American Rheumatism Association; DSM-III, Diagnostic and Statistical Manual of Mental Disorders, 3rd revision; ESR, erythrocyte sedimentation rate; ICD International Classification of Diseases; n.s., not statistically significant; OR, odds ratio; RA, rheumatoid arthritis; s., statistically significant; SMR, standardzed morbidity ratio.

Source: Adapted from Oken and Schulzer (1999) and Eaton *et al.* (1992) and supplemented by our MEDLINE search.

Table 3.37. Hypotheses about the association between schizophrenia and rheumatoid arthritis

Environmental	Pharmacological	Biochemical	Psychosomatic
Institutionalization	Aspirin, salicylate	Histocompatibility factors and other immune-system-related factors	Psychodynamically alternative reactions
Immobility	Analgesic and anti-inflammatory effects of antipsychotic drugs	Excess or deficiency of prostaglandins in schizophrenia and related precursors	Sickest schizophrenics show less psychosomatic disease and the less disturbed schizophrenics show more; chronic
More sedentary and less active life: reduced exposure to trauma in chronic inpatients		Altered serum β-endorphin	hospitalization decreases the prevalence of psychosomatic disorders in schizophrenics
Less exposure to pet cats (Torrey and Yolken 2001)		Altered tryptophan and serotonin metabolism	Reduced tendency or ability to report musculoskeletal pain in schizophrenic patients
Infectious agents		Hyperdopaminergia in schizophrenia leading in some types to a hypoprolactinaemia that might suppress the autoimmune reactions in RA	
		Estrogen dysregulation	
		Altered platelet-activating factor system	

Source: Adapted from Eaton *et al.* (1992), Oken and Schulzer (1999) and Torrey and Yolken (2001) and supplemented by our MEDLINE search.

tolerance, analgesic effects of antipsychotics, or drug and alcohol abuse. The authors called for family studies and genetic research to clarify the multiple hypotheses of the association.

In summary, although the negative association between schizophrenia and RA has been consistently demonstrated and is one of the most striking phenomena in the literature of schizophrenia epidemiology, the reason for the association is as yet unclear. But even if it were due to the mere underreporting of pain by patients with schizophrenia, this would only underline the necessity to look for physical diseases in mentally ill people.

3.18. Nutritional and metabolic diseases

The MEDLINE search on *Nutritional and Metabolic Diseases* yielded 1092 hits. From these, 140 studies were ordered, of which 40 were included. Twelve were added by cross-referencing.

3.18.1. Overweight, obesity, diabetes mellitus and metabolic syndrome

Overweight, diabetes and metabolic syndrome are closely linked. Therefore, the results from the search on *Nutritional and Metabolic Diseases* were combined with studies found in *Endocrine Diseases* and *Digestive System Diseases*.

Not only in the general population, but also in patients with psychiatric disorders overweight, diabetes and metabolic syndrome are a dramatically growing health problem (Mokdad *et al.* 2003). There are currently many research initiatives in this area, studies in progress and a number of new reports are continuously being presented at conferences. It is therefore likely that this part of the review will need to be updated soon. There is a plethora of studies investigating the risk of weight gain, obesity and diabetes associated with different antipsychotic drugs. However, a summary of these studies would go beyond the scope of our manuscript. Therefore the inclusion criteria were restricted to epidemiological studies on the question whether obesity and diabetes are increased in schizophrenia compared to a control group or compared to the general population.

Although not every included study distinguished between each of the following parameters, some important definitions are as follows.

The *prediabetic state* is characterized by *impaired glucose tolerance (IGT)* which is defined as a plasma glucose concentration between 7.8 and 11.1 mmol/l measured 2 hours after a 75-g glucose load. *Impaired fasting glucose (IFG)* is defined as a condition in which the blood sugar level is high (6.1 to 6.9 mmol/l) after an overnight fast, although not high enough to be classified as diabetes

(Zimmet 2005). The diagnosis of *diabetes* is defined by IGT levels >11.1 mmol/l and an IFG level >7.0 mmol/l (Expert Group 2004).

The *body mass index (BMI)*, also known as Quetelet index, is calculated by dividing weight in kilograms by height in metres squared. The BMI does not distinguish between fat and lean mass and is generally not adjusted for age and sex. The normal BMI ranges from 18.6 to 24.9 kg/m^2; *overweight* is defined by a BMI of 25.0–29.9 kg/m^2; *obesity* is classified by a BMI equal to or above 30 kg/m^2 (Coodin 2001).

The *metabolic syndrome*, also known as syndrome X, syndrome X plus, insulin resistance syndrome, dysmetabolic syndrome or the 'deadly quartet', is a cluster of cardiovascular risk factors that occur together in an individual. There are more than six definitions of the metabolic syndrome (Zimmet 2005). A frequently used definition from the Third Adult Treatment Panel (ATP III) includes any three of the following five component risk factors: abdominal obesity (waist circumference >102 cm in men and >88 cm in women), hypertension (>130/85 mm Hg), low high-density lipoprotein cholesterol (HDL-C <40 mg/dl in men, <50 mg/dl in women), elevated fasting serum triglycerides (= 150 mg/dl) and elevated fasting glucose (= 110 mg/dl) (Basu *et al.* 2004).

The prevalence of diabetes has been reported to be about 8% in the United States (Sicree *et al.* 2003). The prevalence is strongly dependent on the geographic region; for example, in Naura, an island in the South Pacific, a prevalence of nearly 30% has been reported (Sicree *et al.* 2003). The latest statistics suggested that 190 million people currently have type II diabetes worldwide and a 72% increase in the overall prevalence of diabetes by 2025 is predicted, with the greatest increases expected in India, China and the United States (Zimmet 2005).

Although the problem of overweight and diabetes in schizophrenia patients has been heavily debated in recent years, a development that is to an important extent due to the introduction of the atypical antipsychotics, we were surprised how few population-based epidemiological studies on the association between schizophrenia and overweight/diabetes exist.

As far back as 1897 Sir Henry Maudsley in *Pathology of Mind* commented that 'Diabetes is a disease which often shows itself in families in which insanity prevails' (Maudsley 1979). Kooy (1919) published the first study on the association between schizophrenia and diabetes. He compared a small sample of ten schizophrenic patients with 20 normal persons and observed elevated blood sugar levels in the schizophrenia group. Numerous studies followed. A summary of 40 epidemiological studies is provided in Table 3.38. Most of these studies focussed on diabetes; overweight was often used as a secondary measure, while only a few studies assessed metabolic syndrome. The quality and design of the reports varied widely and only a very few studies were population based (Dixon *et al.* 2000, McKee *et al.* 1986, Mukherjee *et al.* 1996, Subramaniam *et al.* 2003).

Some important problems are the use of different criteria for schizophrenia and diabetes mellitus (e.g. the 'prediabetic state' was defined only in 1999 by the WHO (World Health Organization 1999)), widely varying publication years (the rates of diabetes have risen in recent decades), small sample sizes, mixing of diagnoses (some studies indicated figures only on psychiatric patients in general), lack of control groups and failure to consider age, gender, ethnicity, geography (thus not taking into account e.g. higher rates of obesity in the United States compared to Europe), medication and diabetes risk factors. Overall, however, the studies showed that overweight and diabetes are increased in schizophrenia. We find it difficult to derive a clear estimation of the excess risk from such a variety of designs, but frequently indicated numbers in other reviews speak of a 1.5–2 times (American Diabetes Association *et al.* 2004) or a 2–4 times higher risk of diabetes than in the general population (Expert Group 2004, Bushe and Holt 2004).

In the current debate of the induction of overweight, diabetes and metabolic syndrome, it is noteworthy that these problems were already prevalent in the pre-atypical area (Dixon *et al.* 2000). A meta-analysis by Allison *et al.* (1999b) showed that the low-potency typical antipsychotics such as chlorpromazine and thioridazine are also associated with weight gain. There are even a few reports, some from the pre-neuroleptic era (Duc 1952, Kooy 1919) and some recent ones on antipsychotically naïve first episode patients (Ryan *et al.* 2003, Thakore *et al.* 2002) suggesting that schizophrenia itself may be associated with diabetes independently of antipsychotic drugs. The theory purporting to explain this association between drug-naïve schizophrenia and diabetes is a dysregulation of the hypothalamic–pituitary–adrenal axis due to psychotic stress leading to hypercortisolaemia and finally diabetes (see Table 3.39). However, due to the small sample sizes in these studies we do not consider the results to be representative (they are hyprothesis generating at best), so that further research on this issue is clearly needed. Other – very plausible – hypotheses on the association between schizophrenia and overweight/diabetes are lifestyle factors (self-neglect, smoking, negative symptoms, lack of exercise, hospitalization, poor diet) and the well-known weight-inducing effect of some antipsychotic drugs (see Table 3.39).

It is clear that the new drugs differ in their propensity to induce weight gain (Allison *et al.* 1999b) and the risk is highest with olanzapine and clozapine. Whether the risk of diabetes differs between compounds is hotly debated, although, given the association of overweight with diabetes in general, it seems plausible that the more weight-gain-inducing antipsychotics would also be associated with a higher diabetes risk (Newcomer 2005). In summary, it needs to be emphasized that the overall epidemiology of overweight, diabetes and metabolic syndrome could be better given the importance of the problem. Further large-scale, population-based epidemiological studies are

Table 3.38. Epidemiological studies on the association between schizophrenia and diabetes, overweight and metabolic syndrome

Study	Country	Research question	Number of patients with Schizophrenia (S) and Control group (C)	Diabetes mellitus (DM), overweight/obesity (O), metabolic syndrome (MS)	Conclusion
Kooy 1919	The Netherlands	Blood sugar levels in patients with dementia praecox compared to normal persons in the Psychiatrische-Neurologische Klinick in Groningen	S: 10 C: 20	DM: Blood sugar levels: S: between 1.01 and 1.33 per mill C: between 0.70 and 1.10 per mill	Slightly elevated blood sugar levels after breakfast in patients with dementia praecox
Duc 1952	Switzerland	Prevalence of glucosuria and diabetes in psychiatric inpatients in the Cery hospital of Lausanne: comparison with Suisse population. Period of observation: 1938–49	Total psychiatric sample: 5991 S: 1667 C: general population of Switzerland	Transitional glucosuria: S: 3.6% All psychiatric patients: 26% C: no data available DM: S: 1.7% All psychiatric patients: 5% C: 1.5%	Elevated transitional glucosuria in schizophrenia patients, especially in the males and in the acute forms. No particularly frequent association between diabetes and mental disorders. Slightly increased prevalence of diabetes in schizophrenia patients
Schwalb et al. 1976	Germany	Prevalence of cardiovascular risk factors in inpatients with different psychiatric disorders from eight different hospitals in Germany	S: 809 C: Organic psychosis: 256 Affective psychosis: 53 Non-psychotic psychopathia: 146 Oligophrenia: 462	DM: S: 19.8% Organic psychosis: 17.2% Affective psychosis: 24.5% Non-psychotic psychopathia: 16.4% Oligophrenia: 15.4%	Higher prevalence of diabetes in patients with schizophrenia and with psychotic disorders than in patients with oligophrenia

Study	Country	Description	Sample	Results	Conclusion
McKee *et al.* 1986	UK	Retrospective study on the prevalence of diabetes in long-stay patients in two psychiatric hospitals in Northern Ireland (Purdysburn Hospital and Downshire Hospital)	Psychiatric inpatients: 2000 C: general population	DM: S: 2.5% C: 1%	Higher percentage of diabetic patients in the examined psychiatric population (2.5%) when compared with the general population data (1%)
Silverstone *et al.* 1988	UK	Prevalence of obesity in outpatients receiving depot antipsychotics from clinics in the City and Hackney Health District in London compared to the prevalence in the general population of London	Psychiatric patients: 226 C: general population	O: Men: Overweight: 39% vs. 33% Obesity: 27% vs. 6% BMI >40: 4% vs. 0% Women: Overweight: 21% vs. 23% Obesity: 31% vs. 8% BMI >40: 6% vs. 1%	The prevalence of clinically relevant obesity was four times that in the general population of Greater London
Mukherjee *et al.* 1996	Italy	Prevalence of diaetes in schizophrenic patients aged 45 to 74 years admitted to a long-term care facility (Ospedale Santa Maria Immacolata, Guidonia)	S: 95 (8 patients off neuroleptics for 1 year, 87 patients with continuous neuroleptic treatment) C: general population	DM: S: 15.8% C: 2.1%	Considerably higher prevalence of diabetes in schizophrenic patients compared to that reported for the general population of Italy. Diabetes more common in patients not receiving neuroleptics for 1 year, no association between diabetes and the use of anticholinergic drugs

Table 3.38. (*cont.*)

Study	Country	Research question	Number of patients with Schizophrenia (S) and Control group (C)	Diabetes mellitus (DM), overweight/obesity (O), metabolic syndrome (MS)	Conclusion
Allison et al. 1999a	USA	Distribution of age-adjusted BMI among individuals with and without schizophrenia. Two data sets: (1) 1989 National Health Interview Survey (NHIS) (2) Schizophrenia patients: baseline BMI data from a drug trial of the antipsychotic ziprasidone supplied by Pfizer Inc.; data source control group: National Health and Nutrition Examination Survey/ NHANES III	(1) S: 150 C: 80130 (2) S: 420 (with ziprasidone treatment) C: 17689	O: (1) BMI men: S: 26.14 C: 25.63 (n.s.) BMI women: S: 27.36 C: 24.50 (s.) (2) BMI men: S: 26.79 C: 26.52 (s.) BMI women: S: 27.29 C: 27.39 (n.s.)	(1) Age-adjusted BMI showed men with schizophrenia have mean BMIs similar to those without schizophrenia. Women with schizophrenia had significantly higher BMIs (2) Minimal, but significant difference in age-adjusted BMI between men and women with schizophrenia compared with the general population

| Brown et al. 1999 | UK | Evaluation of the unhealthy lifestyle of people with schizophrenia living in a community from a 15-year follow-up study and comparison to the general population (Health Survey for England, Bennett et al. 1995)) | Psychiatric patients: 102 S: 39, 22 males, 17 females C: 2291 | O: Overweight (BMI 26–30): S men: 42% C men: 52% (n.s.) S women: 47% C women: 39% (n.s.) Obese (BMI >30): S men: 18% C men: 16% (n.s.) S women: 23% C women: 24% (n.s.) | The prevalence rate of obesity was similar in males, but showed a trend towards an increase in the female schizophrenia patients |
| Dixon et al. 2000 | USA | Prevalence of diabetes in schizophrenia patients (mean age 43 years). Three data sets: (1) Schizophrenia Patient Outcome Research Group – a field study of patient interviews in two states (2) Medicaid data from 1991 from one Southern state (3) Medicare data from disabled persons under 65 and almost all Americans over 65 in 1991. Comparison to the National Health Interview Survey 1994 diabetes rate (Adams and Marano 1995). Period of observation: 1991 | (1) S: 719: 454 men, 265 women (2) S: 6066: 2212 men, 3854 women (3) S: 14 182: 7660 men, 6522 women C: number unknown | (1) DM: Current diabetes: men: 10.8% (s.) women 21.9% (s.) (2) DM: men: 4.3% (s.) women: 15% (s.) (3) DM: men 8.8% (s.) women: 16.7% (s.) C: 1.2% (age 18–44 years), 6.3% (age 45–64 years) | Significantly elevated prevalence of diabetes in schizophrenia patients well before the widespread use of the atypical antipsychotic drugs in the early 1990s. Higher diabetes risk in older people, African–American, Native American and Latino populations, women, lower education levels |

Table 3.38. (*cont.*)

Study	Country	Research question	Number of patients with Schizophrenia (S) and Control group (C)	Diabetes mellitus (DM), overweight/obesity (O), metabolic syndrome (MS)	Conclusion
Coodin 2001	Canada	Comparison of BMI of schizophrenic patients (participating in the Schizophrenia Treatment and Education Program, average age 39.6 years) with the BMI of the general population (results of the Statistics Canada's 1996–7 National Population Health Survey)	S: 183 C: 50 347	O: Average BMI: S: 29.0 vs. C: 25.3 Overweight: S: 28% vs. C: 35% Obesity: S: 42% vs. C: 13.5%	Significantly higher mean BMI in patients with schizophrenia compared to controls
Davidson et al. 2001	Australia	Prevalence of cardiovascular risk factors in outpatients between 18 and 65 years old with mental illness from four Area Mental Health Services in the North-western Health Care Network Mental Health Program in Melbourne. Comparison with the general Australian population (Risk Factor Prevalence Study 1989 and 1995 National Health Survey)	Psychiatric patients: 234 (79% with psychotic disorder, 9% major depressive disorder, 4% bipolar disorder, 3% other disorder) C: general population	O: BMI healthy weight: psychiatric patients: 29.5% vs. C: 49.8% BMI overweight: psychiatric patients: 27.8% vs. C: 22.7% BMI obese: psychiatric patients: 39.7% vs. C: 7.8%	Higher prevalence of overweight in patients with chronic mental illness

Study	Country	Description	Sample	Outcome	Conclusions
Theisen et al. 2001	Germany	Cross-sectional naturalistic study on the prevalence of obesity in inpatients of a German psychiatric rehabilitation centre for adolescents and young adults (mean age: 19.5 years) in relationship to diagnosis and medication regimen	Psychiatric patients: 151 (109 with schizophrenia spectrum disorders) C: Patients with a psychiatric diagnosis other than schizophrenia	O: S: 56% vs. C: 33%	Increased prevalence of obesity among young patients with schizophrenia, especially among patients with chronic atypical antipsychotic treatment
Winkelman 2001	USA	Prevalence of obesity as risk factor for obstructive sleep apnoea in psychiatric inpatients at McLean Hospital, Belmont, MA. Period of observation: 1991–6	S: 46 C: 397 with other psychiatric diagnoses	O: Mean BMI : S: 31.5 vs. C: 27 Overweight: S: 75% vs. C: 52% Obesity: S: 50% vs. C: 27%	Patients with schizophrenia were significantly heavier and had higher rates of sleep apnoea than other psychiatric patients
Homel et al. 2002	USA	Comparison of body mass index levels among schizophrenic versus non-schizophrenic individuals and evaluation of changes in the BMI rates during the decade from 1987 to 1996. Data source: Personal and Characteristic and Health Condition files of the National Health Interview Survey. Method: self-report from a telephone interview	S: 887 C: 427 760	O: Overall mean BMI: S: 27.98 vs. C: 25.74	Significantly higher BMI among schizophrenic patients. Non-schizophrenic individuals showed steady and significant gains in BMI from 1987 to 1996 while schizophrenics showed different time trends. For the most part they showed little or no evidence of an increasing trend in BMI over time. The exception is found among females with schizophrenia aged 18–30 years who showed a dramatically and significantly increased BMI

Table 3.38. (cont.)

Study	Country	Research question	Number of patients with Schizophrenia (S) and Control group (C)	Diabetes mellitus (DM), overweight/obesity (O), metabolic syndrome (MS)	Conclusion
Newcomer et al. 2002	USA	Prevalence of abnormalities in glucose regulation in schizophrenia patients during antipsychotic treatment compared with adiposity and age-matched healthy controls	S: 48 C: 31	O: Mean BMI: S: 27.48 vs. C: 26.26 DM: Mean fasting glucose: S: 87.225 mg/dl vs. C: 74.94 mg/dl	Elevated plasma glucose levels at all time points (oral glucose tolerance test) in the schizophrenia group varying in severity depending on antipsychotic treatment
Regenold et al. 2002[a]	USA	Retrospective, chart-review study on the prevalence of type II diabetes among psychiatric inpatients with various psychiatric diagnoses: schizophrenia, schizoaffective disorder, major depression, bipolar disorders, dementia, aged 50–4 independent of psychotropic drug use at the older adult acute inpatient unit at the University of Maryland Medical Center from 1993 to 1999; Comparison: age-, race- and gender-matched group from the general US population	S: 81 Schizoaffective disorder (SAD): 41 C: general population of USA	DM: S: 13% SAD: 50% C: 15%	Highest diabetes prevalence in schizoaffective disorder at 50%, significantly above the rates expected from national norms. No increased prevalence of diabetes among schizophrenia patients when compared with US population

Thakore et al. 2002	USA	Visceral fat distribution in drug-naïve or drug-free (at least 6 weeks) patients with schizophrenia compared with healthy controls	S: 15 C: 15	O: Mean BMI: S: 26.7 vs. C: 22.8 Intra-abdominal fat: S: 13 323 mm^2 vs. C: 3880 mm^2	Higher BMI in drug-free patients with schizophrenia, similar amounts of total body and subcutaneous fat, but 3.4 times more intra-abdominal fat in patients
Cohen and Gispen-de Wied 2003	The Netherlands	Prevalence of diabetes among inpatients with schizophrenia compared with the Dutch general population	S: 93 C: general population	DM: S: 7.5% vs. C: 1.9%	Significantly higher prevalence of DM among patients with schizophrenia compared to the general population of the Netherlands
Heiskanen et al. 2003	Finland	Prevalence of MS according to National Cholesterol Education Programme in outpatients with long-term schizophrenia from the psychiatric rehabilitation ward at Kuopio University Hospital in Eastern Finland compared to studies in the same geographical area with normal persons. All patients were on antipsychotic medication. Period of observation: Jan–Aug 2001	S: 35 C1: 1038 men (Laaksonen et al. 2002), 204 women (Korhonen et al. 2001) C3a: 207 C3b: 1148	MS: Men: S: 47% vs. C: 1–7% Women: S: 25% vs. C: ~0%	The frequency of MS in schizophrenia patients is two to fourfold higher compared to controls; MS was associated inversely with the daily dose of antipsychotic drugs. No association with any specific type of antipsychotic drug

Table 3.38. (*cont.*)

Study	Country	Research question	Number of patients with Schizophrenia (S) and Control group (C)	Diabetes mellitus (DM), overweight/obesity (O), metabolic syndrome (MS)	Conclusion
McCreadie 2003	UK (Scotland)	Descriptive study on physical health of people with schizophrenia. Assessment by Scottish Health Survey Questionnaire. Comparison of the body mass indexes from patients with schizophrenia living in the community on rural Nithsdale, south-west Scotland, and in urban Partick, west Glasgow, with BMIs from the general population (taken from the Scottish Health Survey 1998)	S: 102: men: 72, women: 30 C: 9047: men: 3941, women: 5106	O: men: S: 70% vs. C: 62% women: S: 86% vs. C: 54%	More patients with schizophrenia were overweight or obese compared to the general population
Ryan *et al.* 2003	USA	Cross-sectional study on the prevalence of impaired fasting glucose tolerance in first episode, drug-naïve patients with	S: 26 C1: 26 C2: GP of three regions in France	Impaired fasting glucose tolerance: S: 15.4% C1: 0%	First-episode, drug-naïve patients with schizophrenia had not statistically significant

		schizophrenia (mean age: 33.6 years). Control: physically healthy Caucasian subjects with no personal or family history of schizophrenia or diabetes mellitus type II (mean age 34.4 years) and comparison of the prevalence of impaired glucose tolerance in a general population study in three regions of France (Gourdy *et al.* 2001)	C2: men: 11.8%, women: 5.2% Mean fasting plasma glucose levels: S: 95.8 mg/dl C1: 88.2 mg/dl Mean plasma level of insulin: S: 9.8 u/ml C1: 7.7 u/ml Mean plasma corticol level: S: 499.4 nmol/l C1: 303.2 nmol/l Insulin resistance (homeostasis model assessment – mean): S: 2.3 C: 1.7	impaired fasting glucose tolerance, higher levels of plasma glucose, insulin and cortisol and were less insulin sensitive than the comparison subjects
Subramaniam *et al.* 2003	Singapore	Chart review on the prevalence of impaired glucose tolerance and diabetes in schizophrenia patients (mean age 55.5 years) from the long-stay wards in Woodbridge Hospital, Singapore, without any atypical neuroleptics compared to the prevalence rates in the general population of Singapore.	S: 194 C: general population Impaired glucose tolerance: S: 30.9% vs. C:15% DM: S: 16% vs. C: 9%	Higher rates of impaired glucose tolerance and diabetes among schizophrenia patients although no patient had received atypical antipsychotics

Table 3.38. (*cont.*)

Study	Country	Research question	Number of patients with Schizophrenia (S) and Control group (C)	Diabetes mellitus (DM), overweight/obesity (O), metabolic syndrome (MS)	Conclusion
Basu *et al.* 2004	USA	Evaluation of the point prevalence of MS in patients with schizoaffective disorder (SAD) – bipolar type (mean age 44.5 years) who participated in an ongoing double-blind study of topiramate or placebo in Pittsburgh, PA	S: 33 C: general population	MS: S: 42.4% vs. C: 24% Mean BMI: S: 37.1 vs. C: 29.1	Of the SAD patients 42.4% met criteria for the point prevalence of MS, nearly double the 24% prevalence rate of the general population in the USA
Cohn *et al.* 2004	Canada	Prevalence of metabolic syndrome in in- and outpatients from the Schizophrenia Program at the Centre for Addiction and Mental Health in Toronto, Ontario compared with rates in the US general population.	S: 240 C: US general population	MS: men: S: 42.6% vs. C: 24% women: S: 48.5% vs. C: 23%	Prevalence rates of metabolic syndrome in patients were approximately two times rates in the US adult population
Enger *et al.* 2004	USA	Comparison of the risks of cardiovascular morbidity in people with schizophrenia with antipsychotic medication in prior 90 days to an index date to risks in age-, sex-, date- and health-plan-matched individuals without schizophrenia. Period of observation : 1995–9	S: treated with any antipsychotic medication: 1920, typical only: 739, atypical only: 562, both: 619 C: 9600	Adjusted RR: New onset diabetes: S: any antipsychotic treatment: 1.75 (s.), typical only: 1.55 (s.), atypical only: 1.52 (n.s.), both: 2.08 (s.) C: 1	Higher rates of new-onset diabetes in patients with schizophrenia than in the general population

Study	Country	Description	Sample	Results	Findings
Hsiao *et al.* 2004	Taiwan	Cross-sectional naturalistic study on the distribution of BMI and prevalence of obesity among Chinese outpatients with schizophrenia treated with antipsychotics. Period of observation: 2002	S: 201: men: 90, women: 111 C: general population of Taiwan (Nutrition and Health Survey in Taiwan 1993–6)	O: Men: Obesity (BMI = 26.4): S: 40% vs. C: 14.6% Severe obesity (BMI = 28.6): S: 23.3.% vs. C: 5% Women: Obesity: S: 39.6% vs. C: 15.8% Severe obesity: S: 27.9% vs. C: 7.9%	The prevalence of obesity among male and female patients was respectively 2.74- and 2.51-fold greater than in the Taiwenese reference population. The prevalence of severe obesity was respectively 4.66- and 3.53-fold greater than that in the Taiwanese reference population
Paton *et al.* 2004	UK	Prevalence of obesity, hyperlipidaemia and smoking in hospitalized patients treated with antipsychotic drugs. Period of observation: 2002–3	S: 166 C: General population of the UK (Primatesta and Hirani 1999)	O: Overweight: 29% Obesity: S: 33% C: men: 18.9%, women: 20.9% Mean BMI: 27.9 Dyslipidaemia: 68%	The prevalence of obesity was almost 50% above population norms
Saari *et al.* 2004	Finland	Serum lipid levels in schizophrenia, comparison with a general population northern Finland 1966 birth cohort at the age of 31 years in 1997	S: 31 C: 5498	Total cholesterol: S: 214.1 vs. C: 196.4 HDL: S: 55.9 vs. C: 60.5 LDL: S: 131.5 vs. C: 116.3 Triglycerides: S: 134.9 vs. C: 104.3 BMI >25 (overweight): S: 58% vs. C: 40%	High lipid levels in subjects with schizophrenia (significantly higher levels of total cholesterol and triglycerides) especially if taking both atypical and typical medication

Table 3.38. (*cont.*)

Study	Country	Research question	Number of patients with Schizophrenia (S) and Control group (C)	Diabetes mellitus (DM), overweight/obesity (O), metabolic syndrome (MS)	Conclusion
Wetterling *et al.* 2004	Germany	Retrospective study on BMI of two samples of schizophrenic inpatients (S1: acute; S2: chronic, over 5 years of treatment) and comparison with BMI data of the German general population. Period of observation: 1998–9	S1 (acute): 90 S2 (chronic): 238 C: German general population	O: S1: mean BMI: 22.3 S2: mean BMI: 25.9 C (mean BMI according to age): 23.0 (under 20 years old), 27.8 (over 56 years old) BMI >30: S1: 1.1% S2: 21.0% C: 11.5%	The bodyweight of first episode schizophrenics is lower compared to the general population. In contrast, chronic schizophrenic patients frequently are overweight or show obesity.
Chafetz *et al.* 2005	USA	Study on the health conditions of patients with schizophrenia or schizoaffective disorder (SAD) compared with patients with other psychiatric diagnoses. Period of observation: 1999–2001	S: 271 C: 510	DM: S: 7.4% vs. C: 3.1 (s.)	Higher prevalence of diabetes in the schizophrenic subgroup. No differences in the proportion of diabetics and non-diabetics who received antipsychotic medication (66.7% vs. 61.2%)

Author, year	Country	Study	Sample	Results	Conclusions
Goff et al. 2005 McEvoy et al. 2005 Meyer et al. 2005	USA	Baseline results on the prevalence of MS in patients with schizophrenia who participated in the Clinical Antipsychotic Trials of Intervention Effectiveness (CATIE) schizophrenia trial and comparison with national estimates from the National Health and Nutrition Survey (NHANES III). Period of observation: 1999–2004	S: 689 C: demographically representative group of the general population (NHANES III)	MS (all): NCEP criteria: 40.9%, AHA criteria: 42.7% MS: Men: CATIE vs. NHANES: 36.0% vs. 19.7% Women: CATIE vs. NHANES: 51.59% vs. 25.1% DM: S: 13% vs. C: 3% (s.) Mean total cholesterol (mg/dl): S: 204.9 vs. C: 204.3 (n.s.) Mean HDL cholesterol (mg/dl): S: 43.7 vs. C: 49.3 (s.)	High prevalence of MS in schizophrenia patients in the USA, especially for women. Schizophrenia patients scored significantly higher on four of the five cardiac risk variables (smoking, diabetes, hypertension, mean total cholesterol, mean HDL cholesterol); only total cholesterol levels were similar between the two groups
Hung et al. 2005	Taiwan	Prevalence of diabetes in patients with schizophrenia (mean age 37.9 years) compared to the general population of Taiwan	S: 246 C: general population of Taiwan	DM: Total: S: 9.8% vs. C: 7.8% (n.s.) 20–29 (years): S: 3.7% vs. C: 1.2% (s.) 30–39 years: S: 6.9% vs. C: 2.0% (s.) 40–49 years: S: 15.9% vs. C: 6.5% (s.) 50–59 years: S: 12.5% vs. C: 25.8% (n.s.) 60–69 years: S: 25.0% vs. C: 25.8% (n.s.)	No significantly different prevalence of DM in patients with schizophrenia from that of the general population of Taiwan Significantly higher prevalence of DM in younger schizophrenic patients (20–49 years) than in the general population, but not in older patients

Table 3.38. (*cont.*)

Study	Country	Research question	Number of patients with Schizophrenia (S) and Control group (C)	Diabetes mellitus (DM), overweight/obesity (O), metabolic syndrome (MS)	Conclusion
McDermott *et al.* 2005	USA	Retrospective review of prevalence of cardiovascular risk factors and frequency of primary care in patients with schizophrenia in comparison with patients without disabilities. Period of observation: 1990–2003	S: 357 C: 2083	DM: Relative risk: S: 1.34 (n.s.) C: no data available O: Relative risk: S: 1.55 (s.) C: no data available	Significantly increased relative risk for obesity in patients with schizophrenia
Ostbye *et al.* 2005	USA	Population-based, retrospective cohort study of outpatients with atypical antipsychotic drugs and the risk of DM compared to patients with traditional antipsychotics, antidepressants, or antibiotics. Period of observation: 2000–2	S: atypical: 10 265, typical: 4607 C: patients with antidepressive medication: 60 856, patients without mental disorder and antibiotic treatment: 59 878	Annual unadjusted incidence rates of diabetes (new cases per 1000 per year): S: atypical: 7.5 vs. typical: 11.3 C: antidepressants: 7.8 vs. antibiotics: 5.1	Higher rates of DM onset in psychiatric patients with antipsychotic or antidepressive treatment compared to the control group with antibiotic treatment, but no higher rate of DM in outpatients taking atypical antipsychotics compared to subjects taking traditional antipsychotics or antidepressants

				MS:	High prevalence of metabolic syndrome in patients with schizophrenia. After controlling for sex, the risk of metabolic syndrome was 3.7
Saari et al. 2005	Finland	Prevalence of metabolic syndrome in the Northern Finland 1966 birth cohort. Study period: 1997–8	S: 31 C: 5455	MS: S: 19.4% vs. C: 6% (s.)	
De Hert et al. 2006	Belgium	Prospective cross-sectional study on the prevalence of MS in patients with schizophrenia treated with antipsychotic medication. Period of observation: 2003–5	S: 430 C: general Belgian population	MS: S: according to ATP -III criteria: 28.4% according to ATP -III A criteria: 32.2% according to IDF: 36% C: 12%	High prevalence of MS among treated patients with schizophrenia. The prevalence of MS is at least twice as high compared to an age-adjusted community sample in Belgium

Table 3.38. (*cont.*)

Study	Country	Research question	Number of patients with Schizophrenia (S) and Control group (C)	Diabetes mellitus (DM), overweight/obesity (O), metabolic syndrome (MS)	Conclusion
Dickerson *et al.* 2006	USA	Study on the distribution of BMI and correlates of BMI in 169 patients with mental illness (96% receiving psychotropic medication) compared with the results of 2404 gender-, age- and race-matched controls from the National Health and Examination Survey (NHANES III) data set. Period of observation: March–December 2000	S: 81 patients with schizophrenia and 88 with major mood disorder C: 2404	Mean BMI: Men: S: 29.0 vs. C: 26.8 Women: S: 32.3 vs. C: 27.2 Obesity: Men: S: 41% vs. C: 20% Women: S: 50% vs. C: 27%	Higher prevalence of obesity in persons with serious mental illness

| Filik et al. 2006 | UK | Prevalence study on the cardiovascular and respiratory health of 602 patients with schizophrenia-related psychoses compared with findings of health surveys of the general population of England in 1995 and 1998. Period of observation: 1999–2002 | S: 482 C: 14 300 | Obesity: S: 34.95% vs. C: 19.4% (s.) | Obesity was more frequent in those with schizophrenic psychoses, and especially in younger age groups |

[a] The study evaluated male and female patients, but numbers are only presented for female patients,

[b] Quoted from Holt et al. (2004), data on control group not available.

AHA, American Heart Association; ATP, Adult Treatment Panel; BMI, body mass index; CATIE, Clinical Trials of Antipsychotic Treatment Effectiveness; DM, diabetes mellitus; HDL, high-density lipoprotein; LDL, low-density lipoprotein; MS, metabolic syndrome; NCEP, National Cholesterol Education Program; n.s., not statistically significant; RR, relative risk; O, overweight/obesity; s., statistically significant; STEP, Schizophrenia Treatment and Education Program.

Table 3.39. Hypotheses on the association between schizophrenia and diabetes

Environmental	Pharmacological	Biochemical	Others
Institutional lifestyle	Weight-inducing and diabetogenic effect of some antipsychotic drugs	Over-excitement of the sympathetic system, hypersecretion of adrenalin	Inefficiency of the liver
Poor health-related behaviour: sedentary lifestyle, smoking, substance abuse, impaired social relationships, economic hardship, inadequate self-care and adherence to prescribed therapies		Dysregulation of the hypothalamic–pituitary–adrenal axis	Positive family history of diabetes (genetic)
Lack of exercise		Hypercortisolaemia, excessive visceral fat, hyperglycaemia, hyperinsulinaemia, insulin resistance	Low birthweight
Adverse diet, poor nutrition, high intake of fast food		Anti-insulin factor	
Lethargy		Abnormal glucose metabolism	
Inadequate medical or public healthcare		Sex hormones and oestradiol mediating weight gain	
General lack of understanding of dietary principles			
Stress of hospitalization			
Psychotic stress			

source: Adapted from Brown *et al.* (1999), Holt *et al.* (2004), Meyer *et al.* (2005) and Zimmet (2005).

warranted. Such studies must be undertaken in different countries, because the risk in the normal populations may differ greatly, e.g. the rates of overweight and diabetes seem to be higher in the United States than in most European countries. Nevertheless, it is clear that the overall risk is increased. Since overweight, metabolic syndrome and diabetes are very serious problems associated with cardiovascular and other deaths, prevention and monitoring of these conditions would appear to be crucial. Guidelines for monitoring have been presented (American Diabetes Association. *et al.* 2006, Marder *et al.* 2004).

3.18.2. Polydipsia

Eight reports dealt with the occurrence of polydipsia and its consequences in schizophrenic patients. Another MEDLINE search on *Polydipsia* was made, which yielded 115 hits. Eight studies were ordered and these eight were included. Four reports were added by cross-referencing.

Polydipsia is a disorder that can have life-threatening consequences. It can pass through three stages (de Leon *et al.* 1994): *simple polydipsia* with accompanying polyuria, conventionally defined as drinking 3 or more litres per day. In extreme cases, polydipsic patients drink up to 15 litres per day, usually water, but also other fluids such as sodas or coffee or even urine. Polydipsia can lead to *water intoxication* with *hyponatraemia*. It can cause neurological symptoms such as nausea, vomiting, delirium, ataxia, seizures and coma, and even death (Vieweg *et al.* 1985).

In chronic water intoxication (e.g. after 5 years) *physical complications* can develop – mainly osteoporosis and dilatation of urinary and gastrointestinal tracts, but cases of cardiac failure, hypertension, malnutrition and others have also been reported.

Hoskins and Sleeper (1933) and Sleeper (1935) already noted an abnormally high urine output among chronic psychiatric patients in the pre-neuroleptic era. A review by de Leon *et al.* (1994) summarized epidemiological studies up to 1994. An update of their review is presented in Table 3.40. Although the results of the individual studies differ substantially, which is at least in part due to varying definitions and measurement methods of polyuria, de Leon *et al.* (1994) concluded that on the whole polydipsia is present in more than 20% of chronic psychiatric inpatients and that this condition might even be underdiagnosed because of difficulties in recognizing this behaviour within the clinical context.

The figures on the prevalence of episodes of *water intoxication* again vary dramatically (0%–80%). As a conservative estimate mainly based on chart reviews which may underestimate the true risk due to difficulties in identifying cases in routine settings, de Leon *et al.* (1994) suggested that at least 5% of chronic inpatients develop the disorder. An analysis only of patients with polydipsia has reported an average prevalence of 29% in single time surveys (de Leon *et al.* 1994).

In terms of risk factors for the disorder, Ferrier (1985) and Riggs *et al.* (1991) found that around 80% of patients with polydipsia and water intoxication had a diagnosis of schizophrenia. Schizophrenia has thus been suggested as a risk factor (Evenson *et al.* 1987), although two studies refuted this assumption by finding no significant differences compared to other psychiatric diagnoses (Emsley *et al.* 1990, Shah and Greenberg 1992). These last three studies did not use reliable diagnostic criteria; hence the question of the effect of the diagnosis remains open. In their 1994 review de Leon *et al.* (1994) summarized that the most frequently reported risk factors were chronicity of the illness, smoking and drugs that decrease the excretion of free water (e.g. carbamazepine, thiazide). Less consistently reported were male gender and white race.

An enormous difficulty in this area is the detection and measurement of polydipsia in psychiatric patients. This difficulty may account to a considerable extent for the high variation of prevalence rates reported above. Generally, polydipsia can be assessed by staff reports and biological measurements of polyuria. Obviously, staff reports may underestimate the prevalence of the problem, because in routine care we usually do not measure how much liquids patients ingest. Biological determinants that have been used are catheterization, 24-hourly urine collection, specific gravity of urine (SPGU) below 1.009, sodium levels and normalized diurnal weight gain (NDWG). De Leon *et al.* (1994) suggested firstly that medical and iatrogenic causes such as diabetes insipidus or medications (e.g. lithium, carbamazepine) should be excluded. After that a combination of clinical and biological determinants should be used because all single methods have their advantages as well as drawbacks (de Leon *et al.* 1994).

The precise mechanism by which psychiatric patients, above all those with a diagnosis of schizophrenia, become polydipsic is unclear. Delusional ideas and hallucinations might cause excessive drinking (Kirch *et al.* 1985). Millson *et al.* (1993) proposed that polydipsia might be an addictive behaviour in which mild overhydration is experienced as pleasurable. Psychiatric medication has been discussed as causing mouth dryness because of its anticholinergic effects, but polydipsic patients had already been reported in the pre-neuroleptic era. There is also a speculation about direct cerebral effects of psychotropic drugs. Dopamine dysfunction, and hypothalamic and hippocampal dysfunction are other hypotheses.

The pathophysiology of water intoxication can be more easily explained by three factors – polydipsia, inability to excrete water (due to kidney dysfunction or abnormal antidiuretic hormone (ADH) release) and reduced sensitivity of the CNS to hyponatraemia (de Leon *et al.* 1994). The physical complications such as osteoporosis are the consequences of these disturbances.

Although studies on polydipsia showed a wide range of different prevalence rates, it seems to be clear that this problem is frequent in chronic psychiatric inpatients and that it is often underdiagnosed. Given methodological limitations of the available studies further research certainly still is warranted from

Table 3.40. Schizophrenia and polydipsia

Study	Country	Method	Number of patients with psychiatric diagnoses (P), schizophrenia (S), control (C)	Polydipsia (PD) (%), polyuria (PU) (%), water intoxication (WI) (%), WI in PD (%)
Jose and Perez-Cruet 1979	USA	Chart review and staff interview on the prevalence of polydipsia/WI/WI in PD in a part sampling of a long-term hospital	P: 239 chronic inpatients	6, 6–3, 350
Blum *et al.* 1983	USA	Staff interview and SPGU on the prevalence of polydipsia in a part sampling of a long-term hospital	P: 234 chronic veterans	17, 5–, –, –
Okura and Morii 1986	Japan	Staff interview on the prevalence of polydipsia/ WI / WI in PD in a long-term hospital	P: 225 chronic inpatients	3, 1–2, 786
Vieweg *et al.* 1986	USA	SPGU (<1.009) on the prevalence of polyuria in a part sampling of a long-term hospital	P: 103 chronic inpatients	–39, 6–
Evenson *et al.* 1987	USA	Chart review and staff report on the prevalence of polydipsia/ WI/WI in PD in a long-term hospital, a mental health centre and a boarding home	P: 2100 in- and outpatients	6, 2–1, 525
Emsley *et al.* 1990	South Africa	Chart review for hyponatraemic patients in a long-term hospital	P: 690 chronic inpatients	–6, 4–

Table 3.40. (cont.)

Study	Country	Method	Number of patients with psychiatric diagnoses (P), schizophrenia (S), control (C)	Polydipsia (PD) (%), polyuria (PU) (%), water intoxication (WI) (%), WI in PD (%)
Peh et al. 1990	Singapore	Chart review for WI in staff identified WI patients in a long-term hospital	P: 2330 chronic inpatients (70.4% with schizophrenia)	−1, 1−
Bremner and Regan 1991	UK	Chart review, staff report and SPGU on the prevalence of polydipsia/ WI/ WI in PD in a hospital for mentally retarded patients	Mentally retarded inpatients: 887	2, 5−1, 026
Shah and Greenberg 1992	USA	Chart review for WI in staff identified WI patients in a long-term hospital	P: 635 chronic inpatients	−4, 9−
de Leon et al. 1996	USA	Cross-sectional survey (chart review, staff report, SPGU, NDWG, clinical interview, DSM-III-R criteria) about the prevalence of polydipsia among inpatients at the Haverford State Hospital. Period of observation: during first week of Feb 1990	Total: 360 inpatients S: 191	26 (84% of them with a diagnosis of schizophrenia ->33) 34 5 52
Chong et al. 1997	Singapore	Case notes reviews (SPGU, NDWG, serum sodium levels) on the prevalence of polydipsia–hyponatraemia among patients with schizophrenia in the long-stay wards of Woodbridge Hospital, Singapore	S: 728	13, 8–13, 6 (1,9 of the schizophrenia population)

Mercier-Guidez and Loas 2000	France	Cross-sectional survey (chart review, ICD-10 diagnostic criteria) about the prevalence of polydipsia in inpatients in one psychiatric hospital and one general hospital in the Somme department of France. Period of observation: during the first week of July 1997	Total: 353 psychiatric inpatients S: 107	10,76 in chronic psychiatric inpatients (42,11 among schizophrenic patients) –18,42 (30,55 were at risk – retrospective chart review)
de Leon et al. 2002	USA	Prevalence of polydipsia (by staff report, SPGU, NDWG) in patients of the Norristown State Hospital, Philadelphia, PA in 1992	Total: 588 psychiatric inpatients S: 449	49 (total sample) /53 (schizophrenia) –4, 4/ 4,7
de Leon 2003	USA	Retrospective review (DSM-IV diagnosis, chart review) about the prevalence of polydipsia in inpatients of a long-term refractory patients at a US psychiatric state hospital. Period of observation: 1996–2000	Total: 61 S: 3229 patients with other psychiatric diagnoses	21 (total sample) /25 (schizophrenia) hyponatraemia: 11(total sample)/13 (schizophrenia)

DSM-111, Diagnostic and Statistical Manual of Mental Disorders, 3rd revision; DSM-IV, Diagnostic and Statistical Manual of Mental Disorders, 4th revision; ICD-10, International Classification of Diseases, 10th revision; NDWG, normalized diurnal weight gain; PD, polydipsia; PU, polyuria; SPGU, specific gravity of urine; WI, water intoxication; WI in PD, water intoxication in polydipsia.

source: Modified from de Leon *et al.* (1994)

both an epidemiological as well as from a pathophysiological point of view. A crucial question is also how often polydipsia leads to serious medical problems, because definitions for 'water intoxication' were often relatively mild, e.g. merely a simple hyponatraemia. Finally, treatments for the disorder also need to be evaluated. Some preliminary studies, e.g. on clozapine, olanzapine, risperidone, irbesartan, antibiotics or opiate antagonists, have been reported, but certainly no recommendable treatment is to date available (Brookes and Ahmed 2002).

3.18.3. Idiopathic unconjugated hyperbilirubinaemia (Gilbert's syndrome)

Muller *et al.* (1991) screened 892 psychiatric patients over the period of 1 year for the incidence of benign hyperbilirubinaemia (Gilbert's syndrome). The incidence of unconjugated, mild, persistent hyperbilirubinaemia in the general population has been reported to be 6–10% and mostly affects males between 20–40 years of age (Taylor 1984). In this study, 11% of the psychiatric patients had increased bilirubin plasma levels. Schizophrenic patients showed a significantly higher incidence of hyperbilirubinaemia (25.4%) than all other diagnostic groups (6.1–9.3%). Müller and colleagues argued against a possible role of antipsychotics to explain the increased rates in schizophrenia.

Miyaoka *et al.* (2000) investigated 290 psychiatric patients over a period of 3 years for the incidence of Gilbert's syndrome. The prevalence in all psychiatric patients was 9.0%, while in schizophrenic patients ($n = 97$) it was as high as 20.6%. This was far higher than the average of the general population in Japan (2.4–7%) (Miyaoka *et al.* 2000). Genetic disposition, an increased vulnerability of red-cell membranes and the role of oestrogen were discussed as possible hypotheses explaining the increased prevalence of Gilbert's syndrome in schizophrenic patients.

3.18.4. Homocystinuria

Bracken and Coll (1985) investigated the association between homocystinuria and schizophrenia. Homocystinuria is an autosomal recessive disorder with an abnormality of methionine metabolism such that methionine accumulates in homocystinuric patients. They found only three cases in the literature in which homocystinuria and schizophrenia coexisted, but reported that there were many other cases of homocystinuria where the patient's mental state was abnormal. They argued that many schizophrenic patients in remission become psychotic when given methionine. As a conclusion they proposed an epidemiological survey to further explore the relationship between the two conditions. According to our review, such a study has not yet been conducted.

Levine *et al.* (2005b) screened plasma homocysteine levels in 193 schizophrenic persons and 762 healthy controls. Homocysteine levels were increased in young male schizophrenic patients compared to healthy controls (mean: 16.3 ± 12 vs. 10.6 ± 3.6). Similar results were observed when they studied serum homocysteine levels in 184 consecutively admitted schizophrenic patients and 305 control subjects. Again, homocysteine levels were markedly increased in this population of newly admitted schizophrenic patients, especially in young male patients.

However, another study by Levine *et al.* (2005a) detected no difference of homocysteine levels in the cerebrospinal fluid (CSF) between schizophrenia patients and controls. Homocysteine in CSF was previously reported to be elevated in a variety of disorders including Alzheimer's disease (Teunissen *et al.* 2002).

In conclusion, there may be a link between schizophrenia and homocystinuria, but the current evidence is inconclusive.

3.19. Endocrine diseases

The MEDLINE search on *Endocrine Diseases* yielded 595 hits; 36 reports were ordered, of which 10 were included. Reports on diabetes, coeliac disease, hyperprolactinaemia, osteoporosis, hyperbilirubinaemia and polydipsia were shifted to other sections.

Studies on thyroid function abnormalities were the only remaining ones that were of interest. Nine reports were added by cross-referencing.

3.19.1. Thyroid function abnormalities

It is well known that both hyperthyroidism and hypothyroidism can cause a number of psychiatric symptoms. The question relevant for our review is, however, the inverse one. How many patients with schizophrenia do have abnormalities of thyroid function?

For a better understanding of Table 3.41, a number of basic thyroid parameters are briefly explained below:

Thyrotropin-releasing hormone (TRH): a hormone produced in the hypothalamus that stimulates the production of thyroid-stimulating hormone in the pituitary gland

Thyroid-stimulating hormone (TSH) or thyrotropin: a hormone produced by the pituitary gland which stimulates the production of thyroid hormones

Triiodothyronine (T_3): the metabolically active hormone produced by the thyroid gland

Thyroxine (T_4): the hormone that is initially released from the thyroid gland; it is peripherally converted to T_3

FT_3I: free triiodothyronine index

FT_4I: free thyroxine index

Table 3.41. Studies on the prevalence of thyroid dysfunction in psychiatric patients

Study	Country	Number of patients with schizophrenia (S), control group (C)	Thyroid dysfunction in psychiatric patients with various psychiatric diagnoses (P), with schizophrenia (S), control (C)
Nicholson et al. 1976	UK	Total: 98 female patients S: 30	Low serum T_4: P: 7 vs. S: 2 Raised serum T_4: P: 1
Rwegellara and Mambwe 1977	Zambia	Total: 478 psychiatric patients	Goitre: All: - women: 34.4%, men: 23.2% Females with affective illness: 57.6% Males with paranoid psychosis: 77.0%
Weinberg and Katzell 1977	USA	Total: 50 psychiatric patients	Endocrine abnormalities (thyroid and adrenal disease): P: 8%
McLarty et al. 1978	UK	Total: 1206 psychiatric patients S: 532	Hypothyroidism: P: 0.5% Hyperthyroidism: P: 0.7% Thyroid dysfunction: P: 1.2%
Cohen and Swigar 1979	USA	Total: 480 newly admitted psychiatric patients	Elevated EFT_4: P: 9% Decreased EFT_4: P: 9%
Levy et al. 1981	USA	150 psychiatric admissions C: 150 patients from a general hospital	Euthyroid sick syndrome: P: 7% vs. C: 7%

Study	Country	Sample	Findings
Morley and Shafer 1982	USA	Total: 386 psychiatric patients Paranoid schizophrenia: 24 Other schizophrenia: 28	Elevated FT_3I: Paranoid S: 25% S other: 7% P (total): 14% Elevated FT_4I: Paranoid S: 21% Other S: 3% P (total): 7.5% Total thyroid abnormalities: Paranoid S: 38% Other S: 10% P (total): 19%
Spratt et al. 1982	USA	Total: 645 acute psychiatric patients S: 258	Elevated T_4: S: 41% vs. P: 33% FT_4I: S: 21% vs. P: 18%
Chopra et al. 1990	USA	Total: 84 hospitalized psychiatric patients C: 84 healthy volunteers	Elevated serum T_4: P: 24% Elevated FT_4I: P: 16% Elevated TSH: P: 17% Suppressed TSH: P: 1% No goitre and antithyroid antibodies

Table 3.41. (*cont.*)

Study	Country	Number of patients with schizophrenia (S), control group (C)	Thyroid dysfunction in psychiatric patients with various psychiatric diagnoses (P), with schizophrenia (S), control (C)
Roca *et al.* 1990	USA	Total: 45 patients with major psychiatric disorders S: 15 C: 53 healthy controls	Significant elevations of one or more thyroid hormone levels: P: 49% C: data not available
Othman *et al.* 1994	Malaysia	S: 249 patients with chronic schizophrenia (136 men, 113 women) C: 601 healthy blood donors (449 men, 152 women)	Thyroid antibodies: Men: S:14% vs. C: 7% (s.) Women: S: 28% vs. C: 13% (s.) Elevated TSH: S: 5% Low TSH: S: 17%
Ryan *et al.* 1994	USA	Total: 269 acute psychiatric patients S: 120	Thyroid disease: P: 3% Euthyroid abnormalities: P: 9.3%
Arce *et al.* 1999	Spain	Total: 172 psychiatric patients	Increased levels of thyroid hormones: P: 30.8% Thyroid disease: P: 5.2%
Sim *et al.* 2002	Singapore	S: 189 inpatients with chronic schizophrenia	Thyroid function test abnormalities: S: 36.4% Clinically euthyroid: all but 1

EFT_4, estimated free thyroxine; FT_3I, free triiodothyronine index; FT_4I, free thyroxine index; T_3, triiodothyronine; T_4, thyroxine; TSH, thyroid-stimulating hormone.

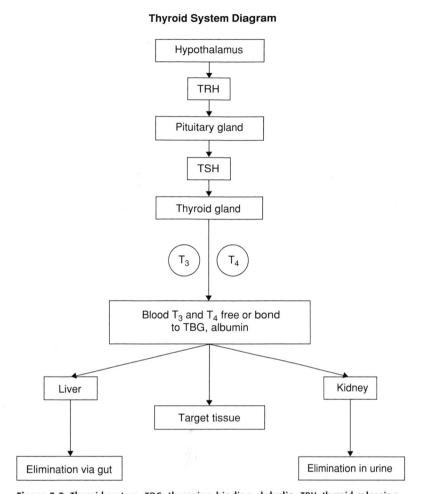

Figure 3.2 Thyroid system. TBG, thyroxine-binding globulin; TRH, thyroid-releasing hormone; TSH, thyroid-stimulating hormone; T_3, triiodothyronine; T_4, thyroxine.

Euthyroid sick syndrome (ESS): elevated or decreased thyroid function tests without clinical thyroid disease which are caused by non-thyroidal diseases

Hypothyroidism: condition characterized by elevated TSH level, low T_3, T_4 and FT_4I

Hyperthyroidism: condition characterized by low TSH level, high T_3, and/ or T_4

The mechanism of the thyroid system is shown in Figure 3.2. In the healthy population feedback mechanisms lead to a reduction of the releasing hormones in the case of too high peripheral thyroid hormones.

The main results of the 14 studies, which will be briefly summarized in the following paragraphs, are presented in Table 3.41.

As thyroid disorders are more common in women, Nicholson *et al.* (1976) measured thyroid function in 98 female patients who were admitted to the acute unit of a psychiatric hospital. Nine females had abnormal T_4 values for different reasons: drug ingestion, recent pregnancy, overt myxoedema. Hypothyroidism was present in four women with non-organic psychiatric disorder. Nicholson and colleagues recommended that female admissions over 40 years of age should be screened for thyroid dysfunction.

Rwegellara and Mambwe (1977) examined 478 indigenous Zambian psychiatric patients who were in hospital on a particular day in January 1976 for the prevalence of goitre. They found that 34.4% of all adult female patients and 23.2% of all adult male patients had goitre, and that 57.6% of all female patients with affective illness and 77.0% of all male patients with paranoid psychosis were found to have goitre. The association between affective illness and paranoid psychosis on the one hand and goitre on the other hand was statistically significant. It is suggested that further work should be done to determine what proportion of patients with depression or paranoia have subclinical or borderline hypothyroidism.

Weinberg and Katzell (1977) determined thyroid and adrenal function in 50 psychiatric patients. Three patients had thyrotoxic symptoms and raised serum thyroid-hormone levels. Psychiatric improvement occurred during remission of the thyrotoxic features. Endocrine abnormalities were found in 8% of the sample. Weinberg and Katzell (1977) emphasized that routine screening is needed to determine the true contribution of thyroid and adrenal disease to psychiatric illness.

McLarty *et al.* (1978) assessed thyroid function in 1206 psychiatric patients. Primary hypothyroidism occurred in five females and one male (0.5%), but in only one patient was the diagnosis clinically obvious. Eight patients were clinically hyperthyroid (0.7%). There was no evidence that phenothiazines or benzodiazepine therapy had any significant effect on thyroid hormone levels. There was a slight difference between psychiatric diagnostic groups; the authors explained this by differences in age distribution.

Cohen and Swigar (1979) screened thyroid function in 480 newly admitted psychiatric patients. Estimated free thyroxine (EFT_4) was elevated in 9% of the cases. In these patients the EFT_4 level became spontaneously normal, usually within a 2-week period, which may be interpreted as an acute 'stress hyperthyroidism'. However, EFT_4 was decreased in 42 patients (9%). In 16 of these patients the level became spontaneously normal. The aetiology of this acute hypothyroidism is unclear. New cases of primary hyperthyroidism and hypothyroidism were low, but a presumptive diagnosis of secondary hypothyroidism was made in eight patients. Nine patients with known thyroid disease were taking inadequate or excessive replacement therapy. The authors recommended thyroid function screening tests in psychiatric patients.

Levy *et al.* (1981) investigated the prevalence of euthyroid sick syndrome (ESS, abnormal concentrations of circulating iodothyronines in euthyroid subjects with non-thyroidal illness (NTI)). They found ESS in 7% of 150 psychiatric admissions as well as in 7% of a general university hospital population. The authors concluded that ESS is as common among psychiatric admissions as in general hospital patients, so that blood thyroid function tests in psychiatric patients should be interpreted with caution.

Spratt *et al.* (1982) measured thyroid function in 645 patients admitted to an acute psychiatric disorders unit. Thyroxine was elevated in 33% (patients with schizophrenia: 41%) and FT_4I was elevated in 18% (patients with schizophrenia: 21%). Serial testing of TRH levels demonstrated both flat and normal responses in patients with a variety of psychiatric diagnoses and at varying stages of thyroid disease activity.

Morley and Shafer (1982) determined the incidence of thyroid abnormalities in psychiatric patients during short-term admissions. Elevated FT_3I and elevated FT_4I were found in 19% of the cases. Elevated test results were particularly common in paranoid schizophrenics (38%). On retesting at 2–3 weeks after hospitalization, the levels of FT_3I and FT_4I had returned to normal in almost every patient. Hypothyroidism was detected in four patients with manic-depressive psychosis. It is warranted to undertake serial sampling to assess the most appropriate time for thyroid function testing after short-term psychiatric admission.

Chopra *et al.* (1990) studied thyroid function in 84 consecutive newly hospitalized psychiatric patients in a 12-week period. Serum T_4 was elevated in 24%, FT_4I in 16%, total T_3 in 20%, FT_3I in 13% and TSH in 17%. Subnormal TSH was found in only 1%. None of the patients with elevated TSH presented goitre or antithyroglobulin or antimicrosomal antibodies. On repeat testing 7–21 days after admission, serum TSH (and/or T_4) normalized in the three of five patients with elevated TSH. In conclusion, in hospitalized psychiatric patients elevated serum T_4 was mainly associated with normal or elevated serum TSH; TSH was suppressed in only 1% of the cases. The transience of high TSH and T_4 and absence of goitre and antithyroidal antibodies suggest that high TSH and T_4 values might be a result of a central abnormality in the CNS–hypothalamothyrotropic axis.

In 45 acutely hospitalized patients with major psychiatric disorders studied by Roca *et al.* (1990), 49% exhibited significant elevations of one or more thyroid hormone levels. The levels of thyroid hormones were correlated with the severity of psychiatric symptomatology.

Othman *et al.* (1994) investigated the thyroid status of 249 patients with chronic schizophrenia. They found a spectrum of thyroid function test abnormalities in chronic schizophrenia. They speculated that this might have been due to an abnormality in the central regulation of the hypothalamo-pituitary-thyroid axis or that the peripheral regulation might be disturbed. However, cases of clinically manifest thyroid disease were rare. They concluded that neither the reasons for the association nor their clinical relevance are clear.

Another study by Ryan *et al.* (1994) performed thyroid function tests in 269 acute psychiatric patients during a 2-year period. Thyroid disease was detected in 3% and euthyroid abnormalities in 9.3%. Ryan and colleagues found lower incidences of thyroid dysfunction test abnormalities in psychiatric patients than some previous reports.

Arce *et al.* (1999) assessed the thyroid status of 172 psychiatric inpatients at the beginning of their hospitalization. They found that 30.8% of the inpatients exhibited abnormal levels of thyroid hormones and 5.2% had thyroid disease. The authors recommended a screening for thyroid disorder in psychiatric inpatients at the beginning of their hospitalization as well as in female patients, schizophrenic patients and patients in treatment with lithium.

Sim *et al.* (2002) performed thyroid function tests on 189 inpatients with chronic schizophrenia. There was a high prevalence of thyroid function test abnormalities (36.4%), but all patients except one were assessed to be clinically euthyroid. No correlation was found between thyroid hormones and neuroleptic use. The authors recommended caution in using and interpreting thyroid function tests in patients with schizophrenia.

In summary, the reports do show high rates of thyroid dysfunction in psychiatric patients. However, these studies are not conclusive nor is their relevance clear. First of all, as in some other section of this book, only four studies (Morley and Shafer 1982, Othman *et al.* 1994, Sim *et al.* 2002, Spratt *et al.* 1982) specifically considered people with schizophrenia; most studies considered psychiatric patients in general. Nevertheless, the studies that examined only patients with schizophrenia also found high rates of thyroid dysfunction. Most studies had no control group. A number of them examined fewer than 100 participants; the largest study included 1206 patients (McLarty *et al.* 1978). Although all studies found abnormal thyroid hormone values, cases with clinically manifest thyroid disease were rare. An exception was the Zambian study by Rwegellara and Mambwe (1977), who found a prevalence of goitre in 77% of the male patients with paranoid psychosis. The prevalence estimates varied substantially in number and type of dysfunction. Both hypo- and hyperthyroidism were present in the study populations. Ryan *et al.* (1994) explained these differences by different study designs and different laboratory techniques. Another explanation was that most of the studies investigated acute psychiatric patients on admission and that the abnormalities were only transient. It is also not clear whether cases of lithium-induced thyroid dysfunction were ruled out by all studies. Levy *et al.* (1981) questioned the increased prevalence, because in their study the values of the psychiatric patients were similar to those in medical patients without non-thyroidal illness: in 150 blood samples of psychiatric admissions there was an incidence of 7% of ESS in psychiatric patients, and this value was identical with the incidence of ESS in the general university hospital population.

Thus, although thyroid dysfunction seems to be frequent in schizophrenia and other psychiatric diagnoses, neither the reason for these dysfunctions nor their clinical relevance is clear. While further research is warranted, new admissions should nevertheless be routinely screened for thyroid dysfunction.

3.19.2. Thyroid cancer

Among the population-based cancer studies summarized in the section on neoplasms (Section 3.4), those of Goldacre *et al.* (2005) and Barak *et al.* (2005) were the only ones to report data on thyroid cancer. There was no statistically significant difference between people with schizophrenia and controls (Goldacre *et al.* (2005)): adjusted rate ratio 0.66, 95% confidence interval 0.08–2.44; Barak *et al.* (2005): standardized incidence ratio 1.02, 95% confidence interval 0.3–.23).

3.20. Immune system diseases

The MEDLINE search on *Immune System Diseases* yielded 594 hits, of which 35 were ordered and only two included in this chapter. The 33 remaining reports were potentially relevant, but they were related to disorders that have been summarized elsewhere in this review (rheumatoid arthritis, HIV and other viral diseases, multiple sclerosis, myasthaenia gravis, hyperglycaemia, coeliac disease, lupus erythematodes, skin diseases). Where appropriate these studies were added to the respective sections.

3.20.1. Autoimmune diseases

One study reported on the association between autoimmune diseases and schizophrenia (Eaton *et al.* 2006). By linking the Danish National Patient Register and the Danish Psychiatric Register they compared 7704 patients having a diagnosis of schizophrenia between 1981 and 1998 with matched controls for the prevalence of autoimmune disease prior to the diagnosis of schizophrenia. A history of autoimmune disease was associated with a 45% increase in the risk of schizophrenia.

Nine autoimmune diseases had a higher lifetime prevalence among schizophrenia patients than among comparison subjects at a 95% level of statistical significance: thyrotoxicosis, intestinal malabsorption, acquired haemolytic anaemia, chronic active hepatitis, interstitial cystitis, alopecia areata, myositis, polymyalgia rheumatica and Sjögren's syndrome.

Five autoimmune disorders appeared more frequently in patients with schizophrenia prior to schizophrenia onset as well as in the patients' parents: thyrotoxicosis, intestinal malabsorption, acquired haemolytic anaemia, interstitital cystitis and Sjögren's syndrome.

The most consistent finding in the area of schizophrenia and autoimmune diseases is the negative relationship with RA. The incidence rate ratio for the schizophrenia patients was very close to 1.0 in this analysis, whereas in most other studies rheumatoid arthritis is much less common in individuals with schizophrenia.

The authors concluded that schizophrenia is associated with a larger range of autoimmune diseases than hitherto suspected. Future research on comorbidity should help in understanding the pathogenesis of both psychiatric and autoimmune disorders.

3.20.2. Allergies

The study by Chafetz *et al.* (2005) who examined the health conditions of 271 patients with schizophrenia or schizoaffective disorder (SAD) compared with 510 patients with other psychiatric diagnoses from short-term residential treatment facilities in San Francisco also reported on allergies. There were no differences in the prevalence of allergies between patients with schizophrenia and patients with other psychiatric diagnoses (2.2% vs. 2.2%).

3.21. Disorders of environmental origin

The MEDLINE search on *Disorders of Environmental Origin* yielded 5385 hits. Despite the enormous number of hits, we found no new topic concerning comorbidity of schizophrenia patients. Some reports have already been discussed in other sections, so no detailed information on the contents of this MeSH term is given.

3.22. Animal diseases

The MEDLINE search on *Animal Diseases* yielded 439 hits. Six studies on the association between Borna virus and schizophrenia were added to the section on virus diseases (section 3.2). Two studies on chlamydial infections and intestinal infections were added to the section on parasitic diseases (section 3.3).

3.23. Pathological conditions, signs and symptoms

The MEDLINE search on *Pathologic Conditions, Signs and Symptoms* yielded 11 955 hits. Despite the enormous number of hits, no new topic concerning comorbidity of schizophrenia patients was found. Some reports have already been discussed in other sections, so no more detailed information on the content of this MeSH term is given.

4

Discussion

Most important findings of the review

The main finding of this review is that there are a number of physical diseases that are more frequent in people with schizophrenia than in the normal population. But there also seem to be a number of medical peculiarities in terms of physical diseases that are less frequent in schizophrenia. A summary of these conditions is provided in Table 4.1.

There were no clearly increased or decreased rates of physical diseases in the categories *Parasitic Diseases, Digestive System Diseases, Otorhinolaryngologic Diseases, Eye Diseases, Hemic and Lymphatic Diseases, Congenital, Hereditary and Neonatal Diseases, Immune System Diseases, Disorders of Environmental Origin, Animal Diseases, Pathologic Conditions, Signs and Symptoms* or these diseases were listed in another category. Please note that physical diseases that have only been shown to be related to the aetiology of schizophrenia (e.g. influenza virus during the pregnancies of mothers of children with schizophrenia) are not listed in Table 4.1.

On the whole, there are some areas that have been studied extensively (for example the comorbidity of neoplasms and schizophrenia for which a number of population-based studies from various countries exist), while other areas are still under-researched. Examples are *Bacterial Infections* and *Virus Diseases*. While mortality studies showed increased mortality due to infections in patients with schizophrenia, the evidence based on comorbidity studies is more limited. With the exception of HIV and, to a lesser extent hepatitis and tuberculosis, there is little evidence on the prevalence of infections in patients with schizophrenia.

Nevertheless, given the enormous amount of research that has been done on physical illness in schizophrenia, neither the health systems nor individual physicians and health institutions have taken consistent and continuous measures to deal adequately with this problem in people with schizophrenia and other mental disorders.

Table 4.1. Summary of physical diseases that occur with increased or decreased frequency in schizophrenia according to our review

MeSH disease category	Physical disease
Bacterial Infections and Mycoses	Tuberculosis ↑
Virus Diseases	HIV ↑↑
	Hepatitis B ↑
	Hepatitis C ↑
Neoplasms	Cancer in general[a] ↓
Musculoskeletal Diseases	Osteoporosis ↑
Stomatognathic Diseases	Poor dental status ↑
Respiratory Tract Diseases	Impaired lung function ↑
Diseases of the Nervous System	Extrapyramidal side-effects of antipsychotic drugs ↑
	Motor signs in antipsychotic-naïve patients ↑
	Altered (reduced) pain sensitivity ↑
Urologic and Male Genital Diseases	Sexual dysfunction ↑
	Prostate cancer ↓
Female Genital Diseases and Pregnancy Complications	Obstetric complications ↑↑
	Sexual dysfunction ↑
	Hyperprolactinaemia-related side-effects of antipsychotics (irregular menses, galactorrhea etc.) ↑
Cardiovascular Diseases	Cardiovascular problems ↑↑
Skin and Connective Tissue Diseases	Skin pigmentation[b] ↑
	Rheumatoid arthritis ↓
Nutritional and Metabolic Diseases	Obesity ↑↑
	Diabetes ↑
	Metabolic syndrome including hyperlipidaemia ↑
	Polydipsia ↑
Endocrine Diseases	Thyroid dysfunction ↑
	Hyperprolactinaemia (side-effect of a number of antipsychotics) ↑

[a] Results on specific forms of cancer were mostly inclusive due to contradictory results and limited power.
[b] A side-effect of chlorpromazine, probably not a problem of most other antipsychotics.
↑↑ Very good evidence for increased risk (e.g. population-based studies).
↑ Good evidence for increased risk.
↓ Good evidence for decreased risk.

Limitations of the review

The following limitations must be considered when reading this review: An enormous number of 44. 567 abstracts was screened using a very broad search strategy that combined the MeSH term for schizophrenia with the MeSH terms of all general disease categories for physical illnesses. This broad search strategy was necessary since there are so many different physical diseases that by looking at individual diseases rather than at broad disease categories we might easily have missed some studies. Although in theory all physical diseases should have been covered by this strategy, this was not necessarily the case because it is possible that the MeSH coding of the papers was imperfect. Indeed, many studies identified by cross-referencing were added to the initial search results. Another limitation is that MEDLINE was the only electronic database used for our review. MEDLINE goes back only to 1966 and does not cover all journals.

Figures 4.1 and 4.2 display the origin of the different epidemiological studies included in this report. They show that most studies (84%) came from North America, Europe and Australia. Only one study originated in Latin America and only two were from Africa, although given the limited healthcare available in theses countries the rates of some comorbid conditions (e.g. HIV in Africa) are probably much higher than in the more developed world, and the frequencies of other diseases such as obesity are probably much lower. Therefore, the results of the review can probably be generalized only to the richer parts of this world. It is possible that further studies have been published in local journals that are not covered by MEDLINE. We would appreciate if readers of this review could send us information on further studies that were missed by our search strategy.

Some of the available evidence on the association between schizophrenia and physical illnesses may be included in studies that looked at serious mental diseases overall rather than specifically at schizophrenia. These studies may have been missed by our search, which combined the MeSH term for schizophrenia only with those of physical diseases. A related problem was that, in point of fact, many studies included in some sections of the review also assessed only serious mental diseases as a whole. The term 'serious mental diseases' implies that many patients had schizophrenia, but it was not possible to disentangle the results on schizophrenia from those on other severe disorders.

We hope that some of the imperfections of the search strategy have been attenuated by cross-referencing of identified studies and review articles and by asking a number of experts in this area about missing studies.

Due to the heterogeneity of the quality and methods applied in the different areas of interest we found it impossible to apply the same inclusion criteria for each category. Some of the areas such as the occurrence of neoplasms in people with schizophrenia have been very well studied, so that we were able to focus on

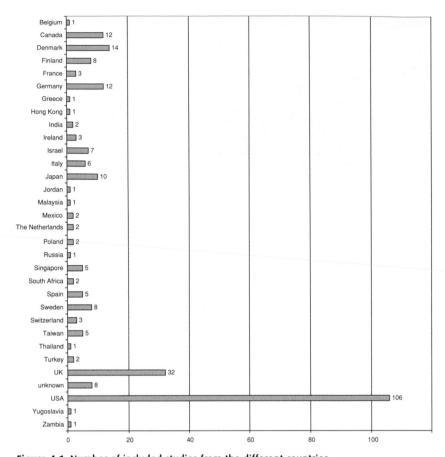

Figure 4.1 Number of included studies from the different countries.

a number of population-based studies. In other areas only a few studies were available, which often did not even include a control group. We included them despite methodological imperfections in order to point to potentially relevant fields and to highlight the need for better studies. For the same reason, meta-analytic calculations were not possible. But we hope that this book can serve as a starting point for meta-analyses in the individual areas.

A general problem was the difficulty of differentiating between simple side-effects of antipsychotic drugs (in which we were not primarily interested) from physical comorbidities proper. Clear definitions are not available. A review of the side-effects of antipsychotic drugs would have gone beyond the scope of this book. For example, weight gain is a side-effect of many antipsychotic drugs, but the resultant obesity and possibly also diabetes are major health problems.

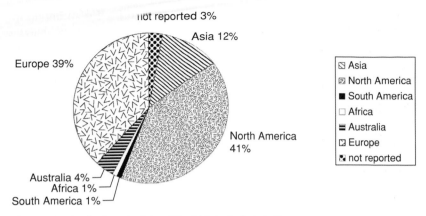

Figure 4.2 Distribution of origin of the 228 included studies

Despite these limitations this review – to our knowledge the first that has covered the epidemiology of the association between schizophrenia and physical illnesses with a broad search strategy – is probably the most comprehensive work on this topic currently available.

Causes for the increased physical comorbidity in patients with schizophrenia

While many specific reasons for increased or decreased rates of physical illnesses in schizophrenia have been mentioned in the specific chapters, the following text provides a more general discussion.

Disease-related factors

One class of factors is related to the changes in the behaviour of people with schizophrenia. Many of them, preoccupied by their psychotic symptoms, may consequently fail to seek treatment. The presence of negative symptoms of schizophrenia such as lack of drive and decreased energy levels may also reduce help-seeking and physical health check-ups. Cognitive disturbance is frequent in schizophrenia and may be another fact that could reduce the patients' communication skills in reporting their problems and managing their medication (Bowie and Harvey 2005, Jeste *et al.* 2003).

People with schizophrenia are often isolated and frequently fail to adhere to the recommendations of their doctors concerning antipsychotic drug treatment, and it can be assumed that they also have problems in maintaining their treatment regimes for physical illnesses (Cramer and Rosenheck 1998).

Patients with schizophrenia have a lifestyle which in itself is an important risk factor for a variety of physical illnesses. According to a recent meta-analysis, 62% of people with schizophrenia smoke, and many of them are using drugs and alcohol (de Leon and Diaz 2005). Although it has been claimed for a very long time that patients with schizophrenia do not exercise much and have poor diets, only very recent evidence has substantiated this claim (Daumit *et al.* 2005, McCreadie 2003).

Factors related to drug treatment

There are also a number of iatrogenic reasons for the excessive comorbidity. Antipsychotic drugs and other medications that patients with schizophrenia must take, usually for many years if not for life, are associated with a number of side-effects such as weight gain, prolactin increase, cardiac effects, motor side-effects and blood dyscrasias, and, we must not forget, can have many untoward drug–drug interactions with other psychotropic and non-psychotropic drugs.

System-related factors and stigmas on mental illnesses

Many people with schizophrenia are unemployed and – depending on the health system of the country they live in – they are often not covered by health insurance (Davidson 2002). There is also evidence that schizophrenia patients have less access to healthcare. Studies have shown that although people with schizophrenia suffer more frequently from cardiovascular problems than the general population, they are prescribed a heart catheterization much less frequently than the general population. People with mental disorders were also reported to be less likely to be placed on HbA1c and cholesterol monitoring, to have a retinal examination to determine whether they have diabetes, to be treated for osteoporosis or to receive medical visits; and they are treated for a physical disease only if it is life threatening (Bishop *et al.* 2004, Cradock-O'Leary *et al.* 2002, Desai *et al.* 2002, Folsom *et al.* 2002, Jones *et al.* 2004, Lawrence et al. 2003, Munck-Jorgensen *et al.* 2000). Once they are hospitalized, adverse events during and after medical and surgical interventions occur more frequently than in persons without schizophrenia (Daumit *et al.* 2006). These problems might have to do in part with the stigma related to mental disorders. The World Psychiatric Association has started a global programme to combat this unsatisfactory situation.[1] The hope is that at the end of this process the physical comorbidities of people with schizophrenia will also be given more attention.

---

[1] See http://www.openthedoors.com.

A problem with many current health systems is also that psychiatry is not integrated into a general medical setting, so that patients with psychiatric problems do not have adequate access to medical treatment. And in many psychiatric centres – especially in the developing world – there is a lack of resources for performing the appropriate laboratory examinations and treatment interventions.

Physician related factors

Last but not least, part of the problem is probably due to the behaviour of the psychiatrists, who often neglect their skills of recognizing and treating physical illness. Sometimes they may consider complaints that are symptomatic of physical illness as an expression of the patient's mental illness and thus miss a medical diagnosis. In the current era of seeking ways to involve general practitioners in the treatment of people with schizophrenia, it will be important for them to become aware of the increased risks of physical illness described above. Doctors in other medical specialties are also often reluctant to treat people with the diagnosis of schizophrenia.

What could be done to change this unsatisfactory situation?

Firstly, we detected a number of areas that have not been sufficiently researched to date from an epidemiological point of view. For example, reviews on excess mortality found that people with schizophrenia die more frequently of bacterial infections, but which infections these are is unclear (Allebeck 1989, Brown *et al.* 2000, Harris and Barraclough 1998). Tuberculosis is an important problem in many parts of the world and it is likely that people with schizophrenia are affected even more frequently. We identified only a few studies on the association between tuberculosis and schizophrenia, although in countries such as Romania special wards for people afflicted with both diseases exist. But more studies are also needed to understand the epidemiological aspects of the relationship between obesity and diabetes in schizophrenia which are enormous problems in the richer countries. It has been stated that the prevalence of diabetes in schizophrenia is 1.5 to 2-fold higher than in the general population (American Diabetes Association *et al.* 2004), but these numbers were not based on a systematic assessment of the available literature, which, according to our review, is heterogeneous and difficult to summarize. Although substantial work has been done in understanding the role played by genetics or antipsychotic drugs in the development of physical diseases, little is known about patient-related factors. There is a general assumption that people with schizophrenia lead a bad lifestyle with little exercise and inappropriate diets that makes them prone to physical illnesses. While this is very clear in the case of smoking, not much evidence is available on other aspects (Daumit *et al.* 2005, McCreadie 2003).

An important area of intervention is that of raising the awareness of physicians in medical specialties other than psychiatry and of general practitioners about the frequent comorbidity between schizophrenia and physical illness. Publications in general medicine journals rather than psychiatric journals could be useful in reaching this goal.

Updating and upgrading psychiatrists' skills of diagnosis and treatment of physical illness is urgent. For example in Germany the curriculum of young doctors specializing in psychiatry includes no practical training in internal medicine. Supplementing the residency programmes by rotations in internal medicine would improve the basic skills of psychiatrists in treating physical illnesses.

Finally, we must combat system-related factors. Stigmatization of mental illness is still widely prevalent. In many countries, most people with schizophrenia do not have health insurance or the means to obtain it. The basic human rights and legal protection of people with mental illness is often neglected, and the conditions in which they live are often terrible. In many countries a significant number of people with mental illness end up in prisons where their somatic complaints are not taken seriously and where they receive no care for them. Psychiatric hospitals and other institutions dealing with mental health problems are often under-equipped and do not have the opportunity to provide necessary clinical examinations and treatments of their patients.

Improving the treatment of somatic illness in people with schizophrenia would make the lives of the people (and their families) who suffer from it more bearable and would save lives – both by reducing mortality from physical illness and by reducing the risk of suicide which for many of them might be the only way to reduce the pain and suffering from their mental and physical illness.

5

Summary

Reviews have established that people with schizophrenia die 15 years younger than the general population on the average. However, unnatural causes (suicide and accidents) account for only 40% of the excess mortality; the rest is due to physical illnesses. While a number of reviews on the excess *mortality* exist, (Brown 1997, Harris and Barrowclough 1998), comprehensive reviews on physical *comorbidities* of people with schizophrenia are not available. Such a review could be important since comorbidity studies examine the risk at a stage when interventions are still possible. We have attempted to fill this gap by providing a review of the association between schizophrenia and physical illnesses using a systematic search strategy.

A MEDLINE search was conducted by combining the MeSH term of schizophrenia with the terms of the 23 general physical disease categories listed by MeSH (first search November 2004, last update May 2006). The search was complemented by cross-referencing of identified studies. Furthermore, a number of experts in the various areas were contacted to obtain information on missing studies. There were no language restrictions. Due to the considerable heterogeneity of the overall study quality in the different areas it was not possible to apply unique inclusion and exclusion criteria. Thus, in well studied areas only population-based, controlled studies were selected, while in other areas studies of lower quality were also included to indicate important future research directions.

The MEDLINE search yielded 44 567 hits. The available data suggest that the prevalence of a number of physical illnesses is increased in schizophrenia. Strong evidence is available for cardiovascular disorders, for obesity and related problems such as diabetes and metabolic syndrome, for obstetric complications and for HIV infections. Although the evidence is not as good as for the former, such problems as tuberculosis, hepatitis B and C, osteoporosis and other problems related to antipsychotic-induced hyperprolactinaemia, poor dental status, impaired lung function, polydipsia, sexual dysfunction and thyroid dysfunction are also more frequent in schizophrenia than in the general population.

Drug-naïve patients often exhibit motor signs which are usually typical for side-effects of antipsychotic drugs, and altered pain sensitivity in schizophrenia has been well documented. But there are also medical peculiarities. A number of large population-based studies suggest that people with schizophrenia suffer less frequently from cancer, and less frequently from rheumatoid arthritis, although this research is not free from potential confounders.

A number of factors probably account for the excess rates of physical diseases in schizophrenia. Some of them are related to schizophrenia itself. Negative and positive symptoms of schizophrenia combined with cognitive dysfunction may lead to self-neglect and poor compliance. Many people with schizophrenia smoke and consume illicit substances. Reduced pain sensitivity probably plays a role. The side-effects of antipsychotic medications such as movement disorders, hyperprolactinaemia and weight gain also contribute to health problems. Many people with schizophrenia are unemployed and are often not covered by health insurance. In terms of system-related factors there is ample evidence that people with schizophrenia have lower access to healthcare concerning a number of medical problems. This situation may have to do in part with the stigmas of mental diseases. Finally, psychiatrists may neglect their skills in recognizing and treating physical illness.

The main strength of the review was the comprehensive literature search. The main limitation was the wide scope leading to an imperfect search strategy. Another major limitation was that 95% of the identified studies originated from industrialized countries. Given the limited healthcare available in developing countries the rates of some comorbid conditions such as infectious diseases may be higher, while others such as obesity and related problems may be lower. Thus, most of the results can not be generalized to developing countries.

Improving the physical health of people with schizophrenia will be a major challenge that requires improvements at various levels. In some areas the epidemiological knowledge must be improved. Antipsychotic medications with fewer side-effects need to be developed. The awareness of patients and doctors must be improved, and there is a need for training of psychiatrists in the detection and treatment of physical diseases. Finally, the system-related causes which have to do in part with the stigma associated with mental illness must be overcome.

References

Abraham, G., Paing, W. W., Kaminski, J., *et al.* (2003) Effects of elevated serum prolactin on bone mineral density and bone metabolism in female patients with schizophrenia: a prospective study. *Am. J. Psychiatry* **160**, 1618–1620.

Adams, P. F., Marano, M. A. (1995) Current estimates for the National Health Interview Survey, 1994. *Vital Health Stat.* **10**, 1–260.

Aizenberg, D., Zemishlany, Z., Dorfman-Etrog, P., Weizman, A. (1995) Sexual dysfunction in male schizophrenic patients. *J. Clin. Psychiatry* **56**, 137–141.

Aleman, A., Kahn, R. S., Selten, J. P. (2003) Sex differences in the risk of schizophrenia: evidence from meta-analysis. *Arch. Gen. Psychiatry* **60**, 565–571.

Allebeck, P. (1989) Schizophrenia: a life-shortening disease. *Schizophr. Bull.* **15**, 81–89.

Allebeck, P., Rodvall, Y., Wistedt, B. (1985) Incidence of rheumatoid arthritis among patients with schizophrenia, affective psychosis and neurosis. *Acta Psychiatr. Scand.* **71**, 615–619.

Allison, D. B., Fontaine, K. R., Heo, M., *et al.* (1999a) The distribution of body mass index among individuals with and without schizophrenia. *J. Clin. Psychiatry* **60**, 215–220.

Allison, D. B., Mentore, J. L., Heo, M., *et al.* (1999b) Antipsychotic-induced weight gain: a comprehensive research synthesis. *Am. J. Psychiatry* **156**, 1686–1696.

Alvarez, L. M., Castillo, S. T., Perez Zuno, J. A., *et al.* (1995) [Activity of aryl sulfatase A enzyme in patients with schizophrenic disorders]. *Rev. Invest. Clin.* **47**, 387–392.

American Diabetes Association (2006) Clinical practice recommendations. *Diabetes Care* **29**. Available online at http://care.diabetesjournals.org/content/vol29/suppl_1/.

American Diabetes Association, American Psychiatric Association, American Association of Clinical Endocrinologists, North American Association for the Study of Obesity (2004) Consensus development conference on antipsychotic drugs and obesity and diabetes. *Diabetes Care* **27**, 596–601.

Apostolakis, M., Kapetanakis, S. (1972) Plasma prolactin activity in patients with galactorrhea after treatment with psychotropic drugs. In *Lactogenic Hormones,* ed. G. E. W. Wolstenholme and J. Knight. Baltimore, MD: Williams and Wilkins, pp. 349–359.

Arce, C. R., Baca-Garcia, E., Diaz-Sastre, C., Baca, B. E. (1999) [Analytical thyroid disturbances in psychiatric inpatients.] *Actas Esp. Psiquiatr.* **27**, 35–42.

Ataya, K., Mercado, A., Kartaginer, J., Abbasi, A., Moghissi, K. S. (1988) Bone density and reproductive hormones in patients with neuroleptic-induced hyperprolactinemia. *Fertil. Steril.* **50**, 876–881.

Atkinson, S. A., Ward, W. E. (2001) Clinical nutrition: 2. The role of nutrition in the prevention and treatment of adult osteoporosis. *Can. Med. Assoc. J.* **165**, 1511–1514.

Ayuso-Mateos, J. L., Montanes, F., Lastra, I., Picazo, d.l.G., Ayuso-Gutierrez, J. L. (1997) HIV infection in psychiatric patients: an unlinked anonymous study. *Br. J. Psychiatry* **170**, 181–185.

Baastrup, P. C., Christiansen, C., Transbol, I. (1980) Calcium metabolism in schizophrenic patients on long-term neuroleptic therapy. *Neuropsychobiology* **6**, 56–59.

Bagedahl-Strindlund, M. (1986) Mentally ill mothers and their children: an epidemiological study of antenatal care consumption, obstetric conditions, and neonatal health. *Acta Psychiatr. Scand.* **74**, 32–40.

Baillargeon, J., Ducate, S., Pulvino, J., *et al.* (2003) The association of psychiatric disorders and HIV infection in the correctional setting. *Ann. Epidemiol.* **13**, 606–612.

Baldwin, J. A. (1979) Schizophrenia and physical disease. *Psychol. Med.* **9**, 611–618.

Ballenger, J. C., Post, R. M., Sternberg, D. E., *et al.* (1979) Headaches after lumbar puncture and insensitivity to pain in psychiatric patients. *N. Engl. J. Med.* **301**, 110.

Ban, T. A., Guy, W., Wilson, W. H. (1985) Neuroleptic-induced skin pigmentation in chronic hospitalized schizophrenic patients. *Can. J. Psychiatry* **30**, 406–408.

Barak, Y., Achiron, A., Mandel, M., Mirecki, I., Aizenberg, D. (2005) Reduced cancer incidence among patients with schizophrenia. *Cancer* **104**, 2817–2821.

Basu, R., Brar, J. S., Chengappa, K. N., *et al.* (2004) The prevalence of the metabolic syndrome in patients with schizoaffective disorder–bipolar subtype. *Bipolar Disord.* **6**, 314–318.

Baxter, D., Appleby, L. (1999) Case register study of suicide risk in mental disorders. *Br. J. Psychiatry* **175**, 322–326.

Beaumont, J. G., Dimond, S. J. (1973) Brain disconnection and schizophrenia. *Br. J. Psychiatry* **123**, 661–662.

Benca, R. M., Obermeyer, W. H., Thisted, R. A., Gillin, J. C. (1992) Sleep and psychiatric disorders: a meta-analysis. *Arch. Gen. Psychiatry* **49**, 651–668.

Bennedsen, B. E. (1998) Adverse pregnancy outcome in schizophrenic women: occurrence and risk factors. *Schizophr. Res.* **33**, 1–26.

Bennedsen, B. E., Mortensen, P. B., Olesen, A. V., Henriksen, T. B. (1999) Preterm birth and intra-uterine growth retardation among children of women with schizophrenia. *Br. J. Psychiatry* **175**, 239–245.

Bennedsen, B. E., Mortensen, P. B., Olesen, A. V., Henriksen, T. B. (2001a) Congenital malformations, stillbirths, and infant deaths among children of women with schizophrenia. *Arch. Gen. Psychiatry* **58**, 674–679.

Bennedsen, B. E., Mortensen, P. B., Olesen, A. V., Henriksen, T. B., Frydenberg, M. (2001b) Obstetric complications in women with schizophrenia. *Schizophr. Res.* **47**, 167–175.

Bennett, N., Dodd, T., Flatley, J., Freeth, S., Bolling, K. (1995) *Health Survey for England 1993.* London: HMSO.

Bergemann, N., Auler, B., Parzer, P., *et al.* (2001) High bone turnover but normal bone mineral density in women with schizophrenia. *Bone* **28**, 248.

Bernstein, L., Ross, R. K. (1993) Endogenous hormones and breast cancer risk. *Epidemiol. Rev.* **15**, 48–65.

Bernstein, L., Ross, R. K., Pike, M. C., Brown, J. B., Henderson, B. E. (1990) Hormone levels in older women: a study of post-menopausal breast cancer patients and healthy population controls. *Br. J. Cancer* **61**, 298–302.

Bilici, M., Cakirbay, H., Guler, M., *et al.* (2002) Classical and atypical neuroleptics, and bone mineral density, in patients with schizophrenia. *Int. J. Neurosci.* **112**, 817–828.

Bishop, J. R., Alexander, B., Lund, B. C., Klepser, T. B. (2004) Osteoporosis screening and treatment in women with schizophrenia: a controlled study. *Pharmacotherapy* **24**, 515–521.

Black, D. W., Winokur, G., Warrack, G. (1985) Suicide in schizophrenia: the Iowa Record Linkage Study. *J. Clin. Psychiatry* **46**, 14–17.

Blackburn, H., Keys, A., Simonson, E., Rautaharju, P., Punsar, S. (1960) Electrocardiogram in population studies. *Circulation* **21**, 1160–1175.

Blank, M. B., Mandell, D. S., Aiken, L., Hadley, T. R. (2002) Co-occurrence of HIV and serious mental illness among Medicaid recipients. *Psychiatr. Serv.* **53**, 868–873.

Bleuler, E. (1911) *Textbook of Psychiatry*. New York: Dover Publications.

Blohmke, M., Koschorrek, B., Stelzer, O. (1970) Hufigkeiten von Risikofaktoren der koronaren Herzkrankheiten in verschiedenen Altersgruppen und sozialen Schichten bei Mnnern. *Z. Geront.* **3**, 201.

Blum, A., Tempey, F. W., Lynch, W. J. (1983) Somatic findings in patients with psychogenic polydipsia. *J. Clin. Psychiatry* **44**, 55–56.

Blumensohn, R., Ringler, D., Eli, I. (2002) Pain perception in patients with schizophrenia. *J. Nerv. Ment. Dis.* **190**, 481–483.

Bonney, W. W., Gupta, S., Hunter, D. R., Arndt, S. (1997) Bladder dysfunction in schizophrenia. *Schizophr. Res.* **25**, 243–249.

Bowie, C. R., Harvey, P. D. (2005) Cognition in schizophrenia: impairments, determinants, and functional importance. *Psychiatr. Clin. North Am.* **28**, 613–633, 626.

Bracken, P., Coll, P. (1985) Homocystinuria and schizophrenia: literature review and case report. *J. Nerv. Ment. Dis.* **173**, 51–55.

Bremner, A. J., Regan, A. (1991) Intoxicated by water: polydipsia and water intoxication in a mental handicap hospital. *Br. J. Psychiatry* **158**, 244–250.

Brookes, G., Ahmed, A. G. (2002) Pharmacological treatments for psychosis-related polydipsia. *Cochrane Database Syst. Rev.* CD003544.

Brown, J. S., Jr. (1996) Geographic correlation of multiple sclerosis with tick-borne diseases. *Mult. Scler.* **1**, 257–261.

Brown, S. (1997) Excess mortality of schizophrenia: a meta-analysis. *Br. J. Psychiatry* **171**, 502–508.

Brown, S., Birtwistle, J., Roe, L., Thompson, C. (1999) The unhealthy lifestyle of people with schizophrenia. *Psychol. Med.* **29**, 697–701.

Brown, S., Inskip, H., Barraclough, B. (2000) Causes of the excess mortality of schizophrenia. *Br. J. Psychiatry* **177**, 212–217.

Bundesgesundheitsministerium der BRD (1991) *Daten des Gesundheitswesens*. Baden-Baden: Nomos.

Burkitt, E. A., Khan, K. (1973) Myasthenia gravis and schizophrenia: a rare combination. *Br. J. Psychiatry* **122**, 735–736.

Bushe, C., Holt, R. (2004) Prevalence of diabetes and impaired glucose tolerance in patients with schizophrenia. *Br. J. Psychiatry* (Suppl.) **47**, S67–S71.

Cadalbert, M., Fenner, A., Schamaun, M. (1970) [Functional megacolon in mental patients.] *Helv. Chir. Acta* **37**, 181–184.

Campbell, E. B., Foley, S. (2004) Coeliac disease and schizophrenia: data do not support hypothesis. *Br. Med. J.* **328**, 1017.

Canuso, C. M., Goldstein, J. M., Wojcik, J., *et al.* (2002) Antipsychotic medication, prolactin elevation, and ovarian function in women with schizophrenia and schizoaffective disorder. *Psychiatr. Res.* **111**, 11–20.

Casadebaig, F., Philippe, A., Guillaud-Bataille, J. M., *et al.* (1997) Schizophrenic patients: physical health and access to somatic care. *Eur. Psychiatry* **12**, 289–293.

Casey, D. E. (1993) Neuroleptic-induced acute extrapyramidal syndromes and tardive dystinesia. *Psychiatr. Clin. North Am.* **16**, 589–610.

Chafetz, L., White, M. C., Collins-Bride, G., Nickens, J. (2005) The poor general health of the severely mentally ill: impact of schizophrenic diagnosis. *Commun. Ment. Health J.* **41**, 169–184.

Chaudhury, S., Chandra, S., Augustine, M. (1994) Prevalence of Australia-antigen (Hbsag) in institutionalized patients with psychosis. *Br. J. Psychiatry* **164**, 542–543.

Chen, C. H. (1994) Seroprevalence of human immunodeficiency virus infection among Chinese psychiatric patients in Taiwan. *Acta Psychiatr. Scand.* **89**, 441–442.

Cheng, H. S., Wang, L. C. (2005) Intestinal parasites may not cause nosocomial infections in psychiatric hospitals. *Parasitol. Res.* **95**, 358–362.

Chong, S. A., Tan, L. L., Wong, M. C., *et al.* (1997) Disordered water homeostasis in Asian patients with schizophrenia. *Aust. N. Z. J. Psychiatry* **31**, 869–873.

Chong, S. A., Mythily, Lum, A., Goh, H. Y., Chan, Y. H. (2003) Prolonged QTc intervals in medicated patients with schizophrenia. *Hum. Psychopharmacol.* **18**, 647–649.

Chopra, I. J., Solomon, D. H., Huang, T. S. (1990) Serum thyrotropin in hospitalized psychiatric patients: evidence for hyperthyrotropinemia as measured by an ultrasensitive thyrotropin assay. *Metabolism* **39**, 538–543.

Cividini, A., Pistorio, A., Regazzetti, A., *et al.* (1997) Hepatitis C virus infection among institutionalized psychiatric patients: a regression analysis of indicators of risk. *J. Hepatol.* **27**, 455–463.

Clarke, D. J., Buckley, M. E. (1989) Familial association of albinism and schizophrenia. *Br. J. Psychiatry* **155**, 551–553.

Clevenger, C. V., Furth, P. A., Hankinson, S. E., Schuler, L. A. (2003) The role of prolactin in mammary carcinoma. *Endocr. Rev.* **24**, 1–27.

Cnattingius, S., Mills, J. L., Yuen, J., Eriksson, O., Salonen, H. (1997) The paradoxical effect of smoking in preeclamptic pregnancies: smoking reduces the incidence but increases the rates of perinatal mortality, abruptio placentae, and intrauterine growth restriction. *Am. J. Obstet. Gynecol.* **177**, 156–161.

Coghlan, R., Lawrence, D., Holman, D'A., Jablensky, A. (2001) *Duty to Care: Physical Illness in People with Mental Illness*. Perth, WA: University of Western Australia, Department of Public Health, Department of Psychiatry and Behavioural Science. Available online at www.populationhealth.uwa.edu.au/dutytocare

Cohen, A. J., Roe, F. J. (2000) Review of risk factors for osteoporosis with particular reference to a possible aetiological role of dietary salt. *Food Chem. Toxicol.* **38**, 237–253.

Cohen, D., Gispen-de Wied, C. C. (2003) [Schizophrenia and diabetes mellitus: not an improbable combination.] *Ned. Tijdschr. Geneeskd.* **147**, 993–996.

Cohen, H., Loewenthal, U., Matar, M., Kotler, M. (2001) [Heart rate variability in schizophrenic patients treated with antipsychotic agents.] *Harefuah* **140**, 1142–7, 1231.

Cohen, K. L., Swigar, M. E. (1979) Thyroid function screening in psychiatric patients. *J. Am. Med. Ass.* **242**, 254–257.

Cohen, M., Dembling, B., Schorling, J. (2002) The association between schizophrenia and cancer: a population-based mortality study. *Schizophr. Res.* **57**, 139–146.

Cohler, B. J., Gallant, D. H., Grunebaum, H. U., Weiss, J. L., Gamer, E. (1975) Pregnancy and birth complications among mentally ill and well mothers and their children. *Soc. Biol.* **22**, 269–278.

Cohn, T., Prud'homme, D., Streiner, D., Kameh, H., Remington, G. (2004) Characterizing coronary heart disease risk in chronic schizophrenia: high prevalence of the metabolic syndrome. *Can. J. Psychiatry* **49**, 753–760.

Colton, C. W., Manderscheid, R. W. (2006) Congruencies in increased mortality rates, years of potential life lost, and causes of death among public mental health clients in eight states. *Prev. Chronic Dis.* **3**, A42.

Conejero-Goldberg, C., Torrey, E. F., Yolken, R. H. (2003) Herpesviruses and *Toxoplasma gondii* in orbital frontal cortex of psychiatric patients. *Schizophr. Res.* **60**, 65–69.

Coodin, S. (2001) Body mass index in persons with schizophrenia. *Can. J. Psychiatry* **46**, 549–555.

Cooper, A. F. (1976) Deafness and psychiatric illness. *Br. J. Psychiatry* **129**, 216–226.

Correll, C. U., Leucht, S., Kane, J. M. (2004) Lower risk for tardive dyskinesia associated with second-generation antipsychotics: a systematic review of 1-year studies. *Am. J. Psychiatry* **161**, 414–425.

Cotran, R. S., Kumar, V., Robbins, S. L. (1989) *Robbins Pathologic Basis of Disease*, 4th edn. Philadelphia, PA: W.B. Saunders.

Council of the National Osteoporosis Foundation (1996) Guidelines for the early detection of osteoporosis and prediction of fracture risk. *S. Afr. Med. J.* **86**, 1113–1116.

Cournos, F., McKinnon, K. (1997) HIV seroprevalence among people with severe mental illness in the United States: a critical review. *Clin. Psychol. Rev.* **17**, 259–269.

Cournos, F., Empfield, M., Horwath, E., *et al.* (1991) HIV seroprevalence among patients admitted to two psychiatric hospitals. *Am. J. Psychiatry* **148**, 1225–1230.

Cournos, F., Horwath, E., Guido, J. R., McKinnon, K., Hopkins, N. (1994) HIV-1 infection at two public psychiatric hospitals in New York City. *AIDS Care* **6**, 443–452.

Cradock-O'Leary, J., Young, A. S., Yano, E. M., Wang, M. M., Lee, M. L. (2002) Use of general medical services by VA patients with psychiatric disorders. *Psychiatr. Serv.* **53**, 874–878.

Cramer, J. A., Rosenheck, R. (1998) Compliance with medication regimens for mental and physical disorders. *Psychiatr. Serv.* **49**, 196–201.

Creese, I., Feinberg, A. P., Snyder, S. H. (1976) Butyrophenone influences on the opiate receptor. *Eur. J. Pharmacol.* **36**, 231–235.

Curkendall, S. M., Mo, J., Glasser, D. B., Rose, S. M., Jones, J. K. (2004) Cardiovascular disease in patients with schizophrenia in Saskatchewan, Canada. *J. Clin. Psychiatry* **65**, 715–720.

Dalton, S. O., Munk, L. T., Mellemkjaer, L., Johansen, C., Mortensen, P. B. (2003) Schizophrenia and the risk for breast cancer. *Schizophr. Res.* **62**, 89–92.

Dalton, S. O., Laursen, T. M., Mellemkjaer, L., Johansen, C., Mortensen, P. B. (2004) Risk for cancer in parents of patients with schizophrenia. *Am. J. Psychiatry* **161**, 903–908.

Dalton, S. O., Mellemkjaer, L., Thomassen, L., Mortensen, P. B., Johansen, C. (2005) Risk for cancer in a cohort of patients hospitalized for schizophrenia in Denmark, 1969–1993. *Schizophr. Res.* **75**, 315–324.

Dasananjali, T. (1994) The prevalence of HIV infection among mentally ill offenders in Thailand. *J. Med. Assoc. Thai.* **77**, 257–260.

Daumit, G. L., Goldberg, R. W., Anthony, C., *et al.* (2005) Physical activity patterns in adults with severe mental illness. *J. Nerv. Ment. Dis.* **193**, 641–646.

Daumit, G. L., Pronovost, P. J., Anthony, C. B., *et al.* (2006) Adverse events during medical and surgical hospitalizations for persons with schizophrenia. *Arch. Gen. Psychiatry* **63**, 267–272.

David, A., Malmberg, A., Lewis, G., Brandt, L., Allebeck, P. (1995) Are there neurological and sensory risk factors for schizophrenia? *Schizophr. Res.* **14**, 247–251.

Davidson, M. (2002) Risk of cardiovascular disease and sudden death in schizophrenia. *J. Clin. Psychiatry* **63** (Suppl. 9), 5–11.

Davidson, S., Judd, F., Jolley, D., *et al.* (2001) Cardiovascular risk factors for people with mental illness. *Aust. N. Z. J. Psychiatry* **35**, 196–202.

Davis, G. C., Buchsbaum, M. S., Naber, D., *et al.* (1982) Altered pain perception and cerebrospinal endorphins in psychiatric illness. *Ann. N. Y. Acad. Sci.* **398**, 366–373.

Davis, J. M., Cole, J. O. (1975) Antipsychotic drugs. In *American Handbook of Psychiatry*, ed. S. Arieti. New York: Basic Books, pp. 441–475.

De Hert, M. A., van Winkel, R., Van Eyck, D., *et al.* (2006) Prevalence of the metabolic syndrome in patients with schizophrenia treated with antipsychotic medication. *Schizophr. Res.* **83**, 87–93.

de Leon, J. (2003) Polydipsia: a study in a long-term psychiatric unit. *Eur. Arch. Psychiatr Clin. Neurosci.* **253**, 37–39.

de Leon, J., Diaz, F. J. (2005) A meta-analysis of worldwide studies demonstrates an association between schizophrenia and tobacco smoking behaviors. *Schizophr. Res.* **76**, 135–157.

de Leon, J., Verghese, C., Tracy, J. I., Josiassen, R. C., Simpson, G. M. (1994) Polydipsia and water intoxication in psychiatric patients: a review of the epidemiological literature. *Biol. Psychiatry* **35**, 408–419.

de Leon, J., Dadvand, M., Canuso, C., *et al.* (1996) Polydipsia and water intoxication in a long-term psychiatric hospital. *Biol. Psychiatry* **40**, 28–34.

de Leon, J., Tracy, J., McCann, E., McGrory, A. (2002) Polydipsia and schizophrenia in a psychiatric hospital: a replication study. *Schizophr. Res.* **57**, 293–301.

De Santis, A., Addolorato, G., Romito, A., *et al.* (1997) Schizophrenic symptoms and SPECT abnormalities in a coeliac patient: regression after a gluten-free diet. *J. Intern. Med.* **242**, 421–423.

Delaplaine, R., Ifabumuyi, O. I., Merskey, H., Zarfas, J. (1978) Significance of pain in psychiatric hospital patients. *Pain* **4**, 361–366.

Delisi, L. E., Smith, S. B., Hamovit, J. R., *et al.* (1986) Herpes simplex virus, cytomegalovirus and Epstein–Barr virus antibody titres in sera from schizophrenic patients. *Psychol. Med.* **16**, 757–763.

Delva, N. J., Crammer, J. L., Jarzylo, S. V., *et al.* (1989) Osteopenia, pathological fractures, and increased urinary calcium excretion in schizophrenic patients with polydipsia. *Biol. Psychiatry* **26**, 781–793.

Desai, M. M., Rosenheck, R. A., Druss, B. G., Perlin, J. B. (2002) Mental disorders and quality of diabetes care in the veterans health administration. *American Journal of Psychiatry* **159**, 1584–1590.

Destounis, N. (1966) The relationship between schizophrenia and toxoplasmosis: *a critical study. Del. Med. J.* **38**, 349–351.

Dewan, M. J., Bick, P. A. (1985) Normal pressure hydrocephalus and psychiatric patients. *Biol. Psychiatry* **20**, 1127–1131.

Dickerson, F. B., Brown, C. H., Kreyenbuhl, J., *et al.* (2004) Sexual and reproductive behaviors among persons with mental illness. *Psychiatr. Serv.* **55**, 1299–1301.

Dickerson, F. B., Brown, C. H., Daumit, G. L., *et al.* (2006) Health status of individuals with serious mental illness. *Schizophr. Bull.* **32**, 584–589.

Dickerson, J. W., Wiryanti, J. (1978) Pellagra and mental disturbance. *Proc. Nutr. Soc.* **37**, 167–171.

Dickson, R. A., Glazer, W. M. (1999) Neuroleptic-induced hyperprolactinemia. *Schizophr. Res.* **35** (Suppl.), S75–S86.

Dixon, L., Haas, G., Weiden, P. J., Sweeney, J., Frances, A. J. (1991) Drug abuse in schizophrenic patients: clinical correlates and reasons for use. *Am. J. Psychiatry* **148**, 224–230.

Dixon, L., Postrado, L., Delahanty, J., Fischer, P. J., Lehman, A. (1999) The association of medical comorbidity in schizophrenia with poor physical and mental health. *J. Nerv. Ment. Dis.* **187**, 496–502.

Dixon, L., Weiden, P., Delahanty, J., *et al.* (2003) Prevalence and correlates of diabetes in national schizophrenia samples. *Schizophr. Bull.* **26**, 903–912.

Dohan, F. C., Grasberger, J. C. (1973) Relapsed schizophrenics: earlier discharge from the hospital after cereal-free, milk-free diet. *Am. J. Psychiatry* **130**, 685–688.

Dohan, F. C., Grasberger, J. C., Lowell, F. M., Johnston, H. T., Jr., Arbegast, A. W. (1969) Relapsed schizophrenics: more rapid improvement on a milk- and cereal-free diet. *Br. J. Psychiatry* **115**, 595–596.

Dorrell, W. (1973) Myasthenia gravis and schizophrenia. *Br. J. Psychiatry* **123**, 249.

Drake, R. E., Wallach, M. A. (1989) Substance abuse among the chronic mentally ill. *Hosp. Commun. Psychiatry* **40**, 1041–1046.

Drake, R. E., Rosenberg, S. D., Mueser, K. T. (1996) Assessing substance use disorder in persons with severe mental illness. *New Dir. Ment. Health Serv.* **70**, 3–17.

Drossman, D. A. (1994) Irritable bowel syndrome. *Gastroenterologist* **2**, 315–326.

Duc, L. (1952) [Contribution to the study of the disorders of carbohydrate metabolism in mental disorders: diabetes and psychoses.] *Schweiz. Arch. Neurol. Psychiatr.* **69**, 89–169.

du Pan, R. M., Muller, C. (1977) [Cancer mortality in patients of psychiatric hospitals.] *Schweiz. Med. Wochenschr.* **107**, 597–604.

Dupont, A., Jensen, O. M., Strmgren, E., Jablensky, A. (1986) Incidence of cancer in patients diagnosed as schizophrenic in Denmark. In *Psychiatric Case Registers in Public Health*, eds. G. H. Ten Horn, R. Giel, W. H. Gulbinat. Amsterdam: Elsevier, pp. 229–239.

Dworkin, R. H. (1994) Pain insensitivity in schizophrenia: a neglected phenomenon and some implications. *Schizophr. Bull.* **20**, 235–248.

Eaton, W. W., Hayward, C., Ram, R. (1992) Schizophrenia and rheumatoid arthritis: a review. *Schizophr. Res.* **6**, 181–192.

Eaton, W. W., Mortensen, P. B., Agerbo, E., *et al.* (2004) Coeliac disease and schizophrenia: population-based case control study with linkage of Danish national registers. *Br. Med. J.* **328**, 438–439.

Eaton, W. W., Byrne, M., Ewald, H., *et al.* (2006) Association of schizophrenia and autoimmune diseases: linkage of Danish national registers. *Am. J. Psychiatry* **163**, 521–528.

Ebert, T., Kotler, M. (2005) Prenatal exposure to influenza and the risk of subsequent development of schizophrenia. *Isr. Med. Assoc. J.* **7**, 35–38.

Ehrentheil, O. F. (1957) Common medical disorders rarely found in psychotic patients. *Am. Med. Assoc. Arch. Neurol. Psychiatry* **77**, 178–186.

Empfield, M., Cournos, F., Meyer, I., *et al.* (1993) HIV seroprevalence among homeless patients admitted to a psychiatric inpatient unit. *Am. J. Psychiatry* **150**, 47–52.

Emsley, R. A., van der Meer, M. H., Aalbers, C., Taljaard, J. J. (1990) Inappropriate antidiuretic state in long-term psychiatric inpatients. *S. Afr. Med. J.* **77**, 307–308.

Enger, C., Weatherby, L., Reynolds, R. F., Glasser, D. B., Walker, A. M. (2004) Serious cardiovascular events and mortality among patients with schizophrenia. *J. Nerv. Ment. Dis.* **192**, 19–27.

Erlenmeyer-Kimling, L. (1968) Mortality rates in the offspring of schizophrenic parents and a physiological advantage hypothesis. *Nature* **220**, 798–800.

Essen-Moller, W. (1935) Untersuchungen ber die Fruchtbarkeit gewisser Gruppen von Geisteskranken. *Acta Psychiatr. Neurol. (Suppl.)* **8**, 1–314.

Evenson, R. C., Jos, C. J., Mallya, A. R. (1987) Prevalence of polydipsia among public psychiatric patients. *Psychol. Rep.* **60**, 803–807.

Ewald, H., Mortensen, P. B., Mors, O. (2001) Decreased risk of acute appendicitis in patients with schizophrenia or manic-depressive psychosis. *Schizophr. Res.* **49**, 287–293.

Expert Group: Schizophrenia and Diabetes 2003 (2004) Expert Consensus Meeting, Dublin, 3–4 October 2003: consensus summary. *Br. J. Psychiatry* (Suppl.) **47**, S112-S114.

Fellerhoff, B., Laumbacher, B., Wank, R. (2005) High risk of schizophrenia and other mental disorders associated with chlamydial infections: hypothesis to combine drug treatment and adoptive immunotherapy. *Med. Hypotheses* **65**, 243–252.

Fenton, W. S. (2000) Prevalence of spontaneous dyskinesia in schizophrenia. *J. Clin. Psychiatry* **61**, 10–14.

Ferrier, I. N. (1985) Water intoxication in patients with psychiatric illness. *Br. Med. J. (Clin. Res. Edn)* **291**, 1594–1596.

Filik, R., Sipos, A., Kehoe, P. G., *et al.* (2006) The cardiovascular and respiratory health of people with schizophrenia. *Acta Psychiatr. Scand.* **113**, 298–305.

Fisher, I. I., Bienskii, A. V., Fedorova, I. V. (1996) Experience in using serological tests in detecting tuberculosis in patients with severe mental pathology. *Probl. Tuberk.* **1**, 19–20.

Folsom, D. P., McCahill, M., Bartels, S., *et al.* (2002) Medical comorbidity and receipt of medical care by older homeless people with schizophrenia or depression. *Psychiatri. Serv.* **53**, 1456–1460.

Fox, B. H., Howell, M. A. (1974) Cancer risk among psychiatric patients: a hypothesis. *Int. J. Epidemiol.* **3**, 207–208.

Freedman, R. (2003) Schizophrenia. *N. Engl. J. Med.* **349**, 1738–1749.

Friedlander, A. H., Marder, S. R. (2002) The psychopathology, medical management and dental implications of schizophrenia. *J. Am. Dent. Assoc.* **133**, 603–610.

Galbraith, D. A., Gordon, B. A., Feleki, V., Gordon, N., Cooper, A. J. (1989) Metachromatic leukodystrophy (MLD) in hospitalized adult schizophrenic patients resistant to drug treatment. *Can. J. Psychiatry* **34**, 299–302.

Gallien, M., Schnetzler, J. P., Morin, J. (1975) [Antinuclear antibodies and lupus due to phenothiazines in 600 hospitalized patients.] *Ann. Med. Psychol. (Paris)* **1**, 237–248.

Geschwind, N. (1977) Insensitivity to pain in psychotic patients. *N. Engl. J. Med.* **296**, 1480.

Ghadirian, A. M., Chouinard, G., Annable, L. (1982) Sexual dysfunction and plasma prolactin levels in neuroleptic-treated schizophrenic outpatients. *J. Nerv. Ment. Dis.* **170**, 463–467.

Gingell, K. H., Darley, J. S., Lengua, C. A., Baddela, P. (1993) Menstrual changes with antipsychotic drugs. *Br. J. Psychiatry* **162**, 127.

Gittleson, N. L., Richardson, T. D. (1973) Myasthenia gravis and schizophrenia: a rare combination. *Br. J. Psychiatry* **122**, 343–344.

Goff, D. C., Sullivan, L. M., McEvoy, J. P., *et al.* (2005) A comparison of ten-year cardiac risk estimates in schizophrenia patients from the CATIE study and matched controls. *Schizophr. Res.* **80**, 45–53.

Goffin, V., Touraine, P., Pichard, C., Bernichtein, S., Kelly, P. A. (1999) Should prolactin be reconsidered as a therapeutic target in human breast cancer? *Mol. Cell. Endocrinol.* **151**, 79–87.

Goldacre, M. J., Kurina, L. M., Yeates, D., Seagroat, V., Gill, L. (2000) Use of large medical databases to study associations between diseases. *Q. J. Med.* **93**, 669–675.

Goldacre, M. J., Kurina, L. M., Wotton, C. J., Yeates, D., Seagroat, V. (2005) Schizophrenia and cancer: an epidemiological study. *Br. J. Psychiatry* **187**, 334–338.

Goldfarb, W. (1958) Pain reactions in a group of institutionalized schizophrenic children. *Am. J. Orthopsychiatry* **28**, 777–785.

Goldman, L. S. (1999) Medical illness in patients with schizophrenia. *J. Clin. Psychiatry* **60** (Suppl. 21), 10–15.

Goodman, S. H., Emory, E. K. (1992) Perinatal complications in births to low socioe-conomic status schizophrenic and depressed women. *J. Abnorm. Psychol.* **101**, 225–229.

Gottesman, I. I., Groome, C. S. (1997) HIV/AIDS risks as a consequence of schizophrenia. *Schizophr. Bull.* **23**, 675–684.

Gourdy, P., Ruidavets, J. B., Ferrieres, J., *et al.* (2001) Prevalence of type 2 diabetes and impaired fasting glucose in the middle-aged population of three French regions: the MONICA study 1995–97. *Diabetes Metab.* **27**, 347–358.

Grady, D., Rubin, S. M., Petitti, D. B., *et al.* (1992) Hormone therapy to prevent disease and prolong life in postmenopausal women. *Ann. Intern. Med.* **117**, 1016–1037.

Grassi, L. (1996) Risk of HIV infection in psychiatrically ill patients. *AIDS Care* **8**, 103–116.

Gregg, D. (1939) The paucity of arthritis among psychotic cases. *Am. J. Psychiatry* **95**, 853–858.

Grinshpoon, A., Barchana, M., Ponizovsky, A., *et al.* (2005) Cancer in schizophrenia: is the risk higher or lower? *Schizophr. Res.* **73**, 333–341.

Gulbinat, W., Dupont, A., Jablensky, A., *et al.* (1992) Cancer incidence of schizophrenic patients: results of record linkage studies in three countries. *Br. J. Psychiatry* (Suppl.) **18**, 75–83.

Gupta, S., Masand, P. S., Kaplan, D., Bhandary, A., Hendricks, S. (1997) The relationship between schizophrenia and irritable bowel syndrome (IBS). *Schizophr. Res.* **23**, 265–268.

Hafner, H., Maurer, K., Loffler, W., *et al.* (1994) The epidemiology of early schizophrenia: influence of age and gender on onset and early course. *Br. J. Psychiatry* (Suppl.) **23**, 29–38.

Halbreich, U., Palter, S. (1996) Accelerated osteoporosis in psychiatric patients: possible pathophysiological processes. *Schizophr. Bull.* **22**, 447–454.

Halbreich, U., Rojansky, N., Palter, S., *et al.* (1995) Decreased bone mineral density in medicated psychiatric patients. *Psychosom. Med.* **57**, 485–491.

Halbreich, U., Kinon, B. J., Gilmore, J. A., Kahn, L. S. (2003) Elevated prolactin levels in patients with schizophrenia: mechanisms and related adverse effects. *Psychoneuroendocrinology* **28** (Suppl. 1), 53–67.

Halonen, P. E., Rimon, R., Arohonka, K., Jantti, V. (1974) Antibody levels to herpes simplex type I, measles and rubella viruses in psychiatric patients. *Br. J. Psychiatry* **125**, 461–465.

Harris, E. C., Barraclough, B. (1998) Excess mortality of mental disorder. *Br. J. Psychiatry* **173**, 11–53.

Harrison, G., Owens, D., Holton, A., Neilson, D., Boot, D. (1988) A prospective study of severe mental disorder in Afro-Caribbean patients. *Psychol. Med.* **18**, 643–657.

Harvey, I., Williams, M., McGuffin, P., Toone, B. K. (1990) The functional psychoses in Afro-Caribbeans. *Br. J. Psychiatry* **157**, 515–522.

Hatta, K., Takahashi, T., Nakamura, H., *et al.* (1998) Abnormal physiological conditions in acute schizophrenic patients on emergency admission: dehydration, hypokalemia, leukocytosis and elevated serum muscle enzymes. *Eur. Arch. Psychiatr. Clin. Neurosci.* **248**, 180–188.

Heiskanen, T., Niskanen, L., Lyytikainen, R., Saarinen, P. I., Hintikka, J. (2003) Metabolic syndrome in patients with schizophrenia. *J. Clin. Psychiatry* **64**, 575–579.

Hennessy, S., Bilker, W. B., Knauss, J. S., *et al.* (2002) Cardiac arrest and ventricular arrhythmia in patients taking antipsychotic drugs: cohort study using administrative data. *Br. Med. J.* **325**, 1070.

Herkert, E. E., Wald, A., Romero, O. (1972) Tuberous sclerosis and schizophrenia. *Dis. Nerv. Syst.* **33**, 439–445.

Herold, G. (2002) *Innere Medizin.* Köln: Gerd Herold.

Hinterhuber, H., Lochenegg, L. (1975) [Gastric ulcers, stress and schizophrenia: incidence of gastric ulcers in male schizophrenic patients.] *Arch. Psychiatr. Nervenkr.* **220**, 335–345.

Hoffer, A. (1970) Pellagra and schizophrenia. *Psychosomatics* **11**, 522–525.

Holt, R. I., Peveler, R. C., Byrne, C. D. (2004) Schizophrenia, the metabolic syndrome and diabetes. *Diabet. Med.* **21**, 515–523.

Homel, P., Casey, D., Allison, D. B. (2002) Changes in body mass index for individuals with and without schizophrenia, 1987–1996. *Schizophr. Res.* **55**, 277–284.

Horrobin, D. F., Ally, A. I., Karmali, R. A., *et al.* (1978) Prostaglandins and schizophrenia: further discussion of the evidence. *Psychol. Med.* **8**, 43–48.

Hoskins, R. G., Sleeper F. H. (1933) Organic functions in schizophrenia. *Arch. Neurol. Psychiat.* **30**, 123–140.

Howard, L., Shah, N., Salmon, M., Appleby, L. (2003) Predictors of social services supervision of babies of mothers with mental illness after admission to a psychiatric mother and baby unit. *Soc. Psychiatry Psychiatr. Epidemiol.* **38**, 450–455.

Howland, R. H. (1990) Schizophrenia and amyotrophic lateral sclerosis. *Compr. Psychiatry* **31**, 327–336.

Hsiao, C. C., Ree, S. C., Chiang, Y. L., Yeh, S. S., Chen, C. K. (2004) Obesity in schizophrenic outpatients receiving antipsychotics in Taiwan. *Psychiatry Clin. Neurosci.* **58**, 403–409.

Hummer, M., Malik, P., Gasser, R. W., *et al.* (2005) Osteoporosis in patients with schizophrenia. *Am. J. Psychiatry* **162**, 162–167.

Hung, C. F., Wu, C. K., Lin, P. Y. (2005) Diabetes mellitus in patients with schizophrenia in Taiwan. *Prog. Neuropsychopharmacol. Biol. Psychiatry* **29**, 523–527.

Hunt, C. E., Shannon, D. C. (1992) Sudden infant death syndrome and sleeping position. *Pediatrics* **90**, 115–118.

Hussar, A. E. (1965) Coronary heart disease in chronic schizophrenic patients: a clinico-pathologic study. *Circulation* **31**, 919–929.

Hussar, A. E. (1968) Peptic ulcer in long-term institutionalized schizophrenic patients. *Psychosom. Med.* **30**, 374–377.

Ingram, D. M., Nottage, E. M., Roberts, A. N. (1990) Prolactin and breast cancer risk. *Med. J. Aust.* **153**, 469–473.

Inoue, H., Hazama, H., Ogura, C., Ichikawa, M., Tamura, T. (1980) Neuroendocrinological study of amenorrhea induced by antipsychotic drugs. *Folia Psychiatr. Neurol. Jap.* **34**, 181.

Jablensky, A. V., Morgan, V., Zubrick, S. R., Bower, C., Yellachich, L. A. (2005) Pregnancy, delivery, and neonatal complications in a population cohort of women with schizophrenia and major affective disorders. *Am. J. Psychiatry* **162**, 79–91.

Jakubaschk, J., Boker, W. (1991) [Disorders of pain perception in schizophrenia.] *Schweiz. Arch. Neurol. Psychiatr.* **142**, 55–76.

Jara-Prado, A., Yescas, P., Sanchez, F. J., *et al.* (2000) Prevalence of acute intermittent porphyria in a Mexican psychiatric population. *Arch. Med. Res.* **31**, 404–408.

Jeste, D. V., Gladsjo, J. A., Lindamer, L. A., Lacro, J. P. (1996) Medical comorbidity in schizophrenia. *Schizophr. Bull.* **22**, 413–430.

Jeste, S. D., Patterson, T. L., Palmer, B. W., *et al.* (2003) Cognitive predictors of medication adherence among middle-aged and older outpatients with schizophrenia. *Schizophr. Res.* **63**, 49–58.

Jones, G. R. (1985) Cancer therapy: phenothiazines in an unexpected role. *Tumori* **71**, 563–569.

Jones, L. E., Clarke, W., Carney, C. P. (2004) Receipt of diabetes services by insured adults with and without claims for mental disorders. *Med. Care* **42**, 1167–1175.

Jose, C. J., Perez-Cruet, J. (1979) Incidence and morbidity of self-induced water intoxication in state mental hospital patients. *Am. J. Psychiatry* **136**, 221–222.

Kaelbling, R., Craig, J. B., Pasamanick, B. (1961) Urinary porphobilinogen: results of screening 2500 psychiatric patients. *Arch. Gen. Psychiatry* **5**, 494–508.

Kales, A., Marusak, C. (1967) Sleep patterns associated with neurological and psychiatric disorders. *Bull. Los Angeles Neurol. Soc.* **32**, 234–242.

Kalkan, A., Ozdarendeli, A., Bulut, Y., *et al.* (2005) Prevalence and genotypic distribution of hepatitis GB-C/HG and TT viruses in blood donors, mentally retarded children and four groups of patients in eastern Anatolia, Turkey. *Jpn. J. Infect. Dis.* **58**, 222–227.

Kaplan, H. S., Sager, C. J., Schwartz, S., Kaye, A., Glass, G. B. (1970) Post-gastrectomy pain and schizophrenia. *Psychosomatics* **11**, 157–163.

Keely, E. J., Reiss, J. P., Drinkwater, D. T., Faiman, C. (1997) Bone mineral density, sex hormones, and long-term use of neuroleptic agents in men. *Endocrinol. Pract.* **3**, 209–213.

Kelly, C., McCreadie, R. G. (1999) Smoking habits, current symptoms, and premorbid characteristics of schizophrenic patients in Nithsdale, Scotland. *Am. J. Psychiatry* **156**, 1751–1757.

Kenkre, A. M., Spadigam, A. E. (2000) Oral health and treatment needs in institutionalized psychiatric inpatients in India. *Indian J. Dent. Res.* **11**, 5–11.

King, D. L., Cooper, S. J., Earle, J. A., *et al.* (1985) A survey of serum antibodies to eight common viruses in psychiatric patients. *Br. J. Psychiatry* **147**, 137–144.

Kirch, D. G., Bigelow, L. B., Weinberger, D. R., Lawson, W. B., Wyatt, R. J. (1985) Polydipsia and chronic hyponatremia in schizophrenic inpatients. *J. Clin. Psychiatry* **46**, 179–181.

Kishimoto, T., Watanabe, K., Takeuchi, H., *et al.* (2005) Bone mineral density measurement in female inpatients with schizophrenia. *Schizophr. Res.* **77**, 113–115.

Kleinberg, D. L., Davis, J. M., de Coster, R., Van Baelen, B., Brecher, M. (1999) Prolactin levels and adverse events in patients treated with risperidone. *J. Clin. Psychopharmacol.* **19**, 57–61.

Klibanski, A., Neer, R. M., Beitins, I. Z., *et al.* (1980) Decreased bone density in hyper-prolactinemic women. *N. Engl. J. Med.* **303**, 1511–1514.

Kooy, F. H. (1919) Hyperglycemia in mental disorders. *Brain* **42**, 214–288.

Korhonen, S., Hippelainen, M., Niskanen, L., Vanhala, M., Saarikoski, S. (2001) Relationship of the metabolic syndrome and obesity to polycystic ovary syndrome: a controlled, population-based study. *Am. J. Obstet. Gynecol.* **184**, 289–296.

Krakowski, A. J., Rydzynski, A., Jarosz, M., Engelsmann, F. (1983) Prevalence of psychosomatic disorders in schizophrenic patients in Poland. In *Psychosomatic Medicine: Theoretical, Clinical and Transcultural Aspects*, eds. A. J. Krakowski, R. Kimbal. New York: Plenum Press, 69–78.

Kroll, J. (2001) Schizophrenia and liver dysfunction. *Med. Hypotheses* **56**, 634–636.

Kunugi, H., Nanko, S., Murray, R. M. (2001) Obstetric complications and schizophrenia: prenatal underdevelopment and subsequent neurodevelopmental impairment. *Br. J. Psychiatry* (Suppl.) **40**, S25–S29.

Laaksonen, D. E., Lakka, H. M., Niskanen, L. K., *et al.* (2002) Metabolic syndrome and development of diabetes mellitus: application and validation of recently suggested definitions of the metabolic syndrome in a prospective cohort study. *Am. J. Epidemiol.* **156**, 1070–1077.

Lambert, M. T., Bjarnason, I., Connelly, J., *et al.* (1989) Small intestine permeability in schizophrenia. *Br. J. Psychiatry* **155**, 619–622.

Lane, E. A., Albee, G. W. (1970) The birth weight of children born to schizophrenic women. *J. Psychol.* **74**, 157–160.

Lauerma, H., Lehtinen, V., Joukamaa, M., *et al.* (1998) Schizophrenia among patients treated for rheumatoid arthritis and appendicitis. *Schizophr. Res.* **29**, 255–261.

Lautenbacher, S., Krieg, J. C. (1994) Pain perception in psychiatric disorders: a review of the literature. *J. Psychiatr. Res.* **28**, 109–122.

Lawrence, D. M., Holman, C. D., Jablensky, A. V., Threlfall, T. J., Fuller, S. A. (2000) Excess cancer mortality in Western Australian psychiatric patients due to higher case fatality rates. *Acta Psychiatr. Scand.* **101**, 382–388.

Lawrence, D. M., Jablensky, A. V., Holman, C. D. J. (2001) *Duty to Care: Physical Illness in People with Mental Illness.* Available online at http://cdh.curtin.edu.au/ publications/2001.cfm/

Lawrence, D. M., Holman, C. D., Jablensky, A. V., Hobbs, M. S. (2003) Death rate from ischaemic heart disease in Western Australian psychiatric patients 1980–1998. *Br. J. Psychiatry* **182**, 31–36.

Lee, H. K., Travin, S., Bluestone, H. (1992) HIV-1 in inpatients. *Hosp. Commun. Psychiatry* **43**, 181–182.

Leucht, S. M., Pitschel-Walz, G., Abraham, D., Kissling, W. (1999) Efficacy and extrapyramidal side-effects of the new antipsychotics olanzapine, quetiapine, risperidone, and sertindole compared to conventional antipsychotics and placebo: a meta-analysis or randomized controlled trials. *Schizophr. Res.* **35**, 51–68.

Levine, J., Agam, G., Sela, B. A., *et al.* (2005a) CSF homocysteine is not elevated in schizophrenia. *J. Neur. Transm.* **112**, 297–302.

Levine, J., Sela, B. A., Osher, Y., Belmaker, R. H. (2005b) High homocysteine serum levels in young male schizophrenia and bipolar patients and in an animal model. *Prog. Neuropsychopharmacol. Biol. Psychiatry* **29**, 1181–1191.

Levy, D. L., Holzman, P. S., Proctor, L. R. (1983) Vestibular dysfunction and psychopathology. *Schizophr. Bull.* **9**, 383–438.

Levy, R. P., Jensen, J. B., Laus, V. G., Agle, D. P., Engel, I. M. (1981) Serum thyroid hormone abnormalities in psychiatric disease. *Metabolism* **30**, 1060–1064.

Lewis, S., Jagger, R. G., Treasure, E. (2001) The oral health of psychiatric in-patients in South Wales. *Spec. Care Dentist.* **21**, 182–186.

Lichtermann, D., Ekelund, J., Pukkala, E., Tanskanen, A., Lonnqvist, J. (2001) Incidence of cancer among persons with schizophrenia and their relatives. *Arch. Gen. Psychiatry* **58**, 573–578.

Lieberman, A. L. (1955) Painless myocardial infarction in psychotic patients. *Geriatrics* **10**, 579–580.

Lin, C. C., Bai, Y. M., Chen, J. Y., Lin, C. Y., Lan, T. H. (1999) A retrospective study of clozapine and urinary incontinence in Chinese in-patients. *Acta Psychiatr. Scand.* **100**, 158–161.

Liu-Seifert, H., Kinon, B. J., Ahl, J., Lamberson, S. (2004) Osteopenia associated with increased prolactin and aging in psychiatric patients treated with prolactin-elevating antipsychotics. *Ann. N. Y. Acad. Sci.* **1032**, 297–298.

Llovera, M., Pichard, C., Bernichtein, S., *et al.* (2000) Human prolactin (hPRL) antagonists inhibit hPRL-activated signaling pathways involved in breast cancer cell proliferation. *Oncogene* **19**, 4695–4705.

Lovett Doust, J. W. (1980) Sinus tachycardia and abnormal cardiac rate variation in schizophrenia. *Neuropsychobiology* **6**, 305–312.

Lycke, E., Norrby, R., Roos, B. E. (1974) A serological study on mentally ill patients with particular reference to the prevalence of herpes virus infections. *Br. J. Psychiatry* **124**, 273–279.

Macdonald, S., Halliday, J., MacEwan, T., *et al.* (2003) Nithsdale Schizophrenia Surveys 24: sexual dysfunction – case-control study. *Br. J. Psychiatry* **182**, 50–56.

Magharious, W., Goff, D. C., Amico, E. (1998) Relationship of gender and menstrual status to symptoms and medication side effects in patients with schizophrenia. *Psychiatr. Res.* **77**, 159–166.

Marchand Walter, E. (1955) Occurrence of painless myocardial infarction in psychotic patients. *N. Engl. J. Med.* **253**, 51–55.

Marchand Walter, E., Sarota, B., Marble, H. C., *et al.* (1959) Occurrence of painless acute surgical disorders in psychotic patients. *N. Engl. J. Med.* **260**, 580–585.

Marcus, J., Auerbach, J., Wilkinson, L., Burack, C. M. (1981) Infants at risk for schizophrenia: the Jerusalem Infant Development Study. *Arch. Gen. Psychiatry* **38**, 703–713.

Marder, S. R., Essock, S. M., Miller, A. L., *et al.* (2004) Physical health monitoring of patients with schizophrenia. *Am. J. Psychiatry* **161**, 1334–1349.

Martinez-Bermejo, A., Polanco, I. (2002) [Neuropsychological changes in coeliac disease.] *Rev. Neurol.* **34** (Suppl. 1), S24–S33.

Mason, P. R., Winton, F. E. (1995) Ear disease and schizophrenia: a case-control study. *Acta Psychiatr. Scand.* **91**, 217–221.

Masterson, E., O'Shea, B. (1984) Smoking and malignancy in schizophrenia. *Br. J. Psychiatry* **145**, 429–432.

Maudsley, H. (1979) *The Pathology of Mind*, 3rd end. London: Macmillan.

May, P. R. A. (1948) Pupillary abnormalities in schizophrenia and during muscular effort. *J. Ment. Sci.* **94**, 89–98.

McCreadie, R. G. (2003) Diet, smoking and cardiovascular risk in people with schizophrenia: descriptive study. *Br. J. Psychiatry* **183**, 534–539.

McCreadie, R. G., Stevens, H., Henderson, J., *et al.* (2004) The dental health of people with schizophrenia. *Acta Psychiatr. Scand.* **110**, 306–310.

McDermott, S., Moran, R., Platt, T., *et al.* (2005) Heart disease, schizophrenia, and affective psychoses: epidemiology of risk in primary care. *Commun. Ment. Health J.* **41**, 747–755.

McEvoy, J. P., Meyer, J. M., Goff, D. C., *et al.* (2005) Prevalence of the metabolic syndrome in patients with schizophrenia: baseline results from the Clinical Antipsychotic Trials of Intervention Effectiveness (CATIE) schizophrenia trial and comparison with national estimates from NHANES III. *Schizophr. Res.* **80**, 19–32.

McGuffin, P., Gardiner, P., Swinburne, L. M. (1981) Schizophrenia, celiac disease, and antibodies to food. *Biol. Psychiatry* **16**, 281–285.

McKee, H. A., D'Arcy, P. F., Wilson, P. J. (1986) Diabetes and schizophrenia: a preliminary study. *J. Clin. Hosp. Pharm.* **11**, 297–299.

McLarty, D. G., Ratcliffe, W. A., Ratcliffe, J. G., Shimmins, J. G., Goldberg, A. (1978) A study of thyroid function in psychiatric in-patients. *Br. J. Psychiatry* **133**, 211–218.

McNeil, T. F., Kaij, L. (1973) Obstetric complications and physical size of offspring of schizophrenic, schizophrenic-like, and control mothers. *Br. J. Psychiatry* **123**, 341–348.

McNeil, T. F., Kaij, L., Malmquist-Larsson, A., *et al.* (1983) Offspring of women with nonorganic psychoses: development of a longitudinal study of children at high risk. *Acta Psychiatr. Scand.* **68**, 234–250.

Meaney, A. M., O'Keane, V. (2002) Prolactin and schizophrenia: clinical consequences of hyperprolactinaemia. *Life Sci.* **71**, 979–992.

Meaney, A. M., Smith, S., Howes, O. D., *et al.* (2004) Effects of long-term prolactin-raising antipsychotic medication on bone mineral density in patients with schizophrenia. *Br. J. Psychiatry* **184**, 503–508.

Mednick, S. A., Mura, E., Schulsinger, F., Mednick, B. (1971) Perinatal conditions and infant development in children with schizophrenic parents. *Soc. Biol.* **18**, S103–S113.

Mellsop, G. W., Koadlow, L., Syme, J., Whittingham, S. (1974) Absence of rheumatoid arthritis in schizophrenia. *Aust. N. Z. J. Med.* **4**, 247–252.

Meltzer, H. Y. (1976) Serum creatine phosphokinase in schizophrenia. *Am. J. Psychiatry* **133**, 192–197.

Meltzer, H. Y., Davidson, M., Glassman, A. H., Vieweg, W. V. (2002) Assessing cardio-vascular risks versus clinical benefits of atypical antipsychotic drug treatment. *J. Clin. Psychiatry* **63** (Suppl. 9), 25–29.

Mercier-Guidez, E., Loas, G. (2000) Polydipsia and water intoxication in 353 psychiatric inpatients: an epidemiological and psychopathological study. *Eur. Psychiatry* **15**, 306–311.

Meyer, J. M. (2003) Cardiovascular illness and hyperlipidemia in patients with schizophrenia. In *Medical Illness and Schizophrenia*, eds. J. M. Meyer, H. A. Nasrallah. Washington, DC: American Psychiatric Publishing, pp. 53–80.

Meyer, J. M., Koro, C. E. (2004) The effects of antipsychotic therapy on serum lipids: a comprehensive review. *Schizophr. Res.* **70**, 1–17.

Meyer, J. M., Nasrallah, H. A. (eds.) (2003) *Medical illness and schizophrenia.* Washington, DC: American Psychiatric Publishing.

Meyer, I., McKinnon, K., Cournos, F., *et al.* (1993) (HIV seroprevalence among long-stay patients in a state psychiatric hospital. *Hosp. Commun. Psychiatry* **44**, 282–284.

Meyer, J. M., Koro, C. E., L'Italien, G. J. (2005) The metabolic syndrome and schizophrenia: a review. *Int. Rev. Psychiatry* **17**, 173–180.

Miller, L. J., Finnerty, M. (1996) Sexuality, pregnancy, and childrearing among women with schizophrenia-spectrum disorders. *Psychiatr. Serv.* **47**, 502–506.

Millson, R. C., Smith, A. P., Koczapski, A. B., *et al.* (1993) Self-induced water intoxication treated with group psychotherapy. *Am. J. Psychiatry* **150**, 825–826.

Mirdal, G. K., Mednick, S. A., Schulsinger, F., Fuchs, F. (1974) Perinatal complications in children of schizophrenic mothers. *Acta Psychiatr. Scand.* **50**, 553–568.

Miyaoka, T., Seno, H., Itoga, M., *et al.* (2000) Schizophrenia-associated idiopathic unconjugated hyperbilirubinemia (Gilbert's syndrome). *J. Clin. Psychiatry* **61**, 868–871.

Modrzewska, K. (1980) The offspring of schizophrenic parents in a North Swedish isolate. *Clin. Genet.* **17**, 191–201.

Mohamed, S. N., Merskey, H., Kazarian, S., Disney, T. F. (1982) An investigation of the possible inverse relationships between the occurrence of rheumatoid arthritis, osteoarthritis and schizophrenia. *Can. J. Psychiatry* **27**, 381–383.

Mokdad, A. H., Ford, E. S., Bowman, B. A., *et al.* (2003) Prevalence of obesity, diabetes, and obesity-related health risk factors, 2001. *J. Am. Med. Assoc.* **289**, 76–79.

Monti, J. M., Monti, D. (2004) Sleep in schizophrenia patients and the effects of antipsychotic drugs. *Sleep Med. Rev.* **8**, 133–148.

Morley, J. E., Shafer, R. B. (1982) Thyroid function screening in new psychiatric admissions. *Arch. Intern. Med.* **142**, 591–593.

Mors, O., Mortensen, P. B., Ewald, H. (1999) A population-based register study of the association between schizophrenia and rheumatoid arthritis. *Schizophr. Res.* **40**, 67–74.

Mortensen, P. B. (1987) Neuroleptic treatment and other factors modifying cancer risk in schizophrenic patients. *Acta Psychiatr. Scand.* **75**, 585–590.

Mortensen, P. B. (1989) The incidence of cancer in schizophrenic patients. *J. Epidemiol. Commun. Health* **43**, 43–47.

Mortensen, P. B. (1992) Neuroleptic medication and reduced risk of prostate cancer in schizophrenic patients. *Acta Psychiatr. Scand.* **85**, 390–393.

Mortensen, P. B. (1994) The occurrence of cancer in first admitted schizophrenic patients. *Schizophr. Res.* **12**, 185–194.

Mukherjee, S., Decina, P., Bocola, V., Saraceni, F., Scapicchio, P. L. (1996) Diabetes mellitus in schizophrenic patients. *Compr. Psychiatry* **37**, 68–73.

Muller, N., Schiller, P., Ackenheil, M. (1991) Coincidence of schizophrenia and hyperbilirubinemia. *Pharmacopsychiatry* **24**, 225–228.

Munck-Jorgensen, P., Mors, O., Mortensen, P. B., Ewald, H. (2000) The schizophrenic patient in the somatic hospital. *Acta Psychiatr. Scand.* (Suppl.) **102**, 96–99.

Muntjewerff, J. W., Blom, H. J. (2005) Aberrant folate status in schizophrenic patients: what is the evidence? *Prog. Neuropsychopharmacol. Biol. Psychiatry* **29**, 1133–1139.

Murphy, G. M., Jr., Lim, K. O., Wieneke, M., *et al.* (1998) No neuropathologic evidence for an increased frequency of Alzheimer's disease among elderly schizophrenics. *Biol. Psychiatry* **43**, 205–209.

Naber, D., Pajonk, F. G., Perro, C., Lohmer, B. (1994) Human immunodeficiency virus antibody test and seroprevalence in psychiatric patients. *Acta Psychiatr. Scand.* **89**, 358–361.

Naidoo, U., Goff, D. C., Klibanski, A. (2003) Hyperprolactinemia and bone mineral density: the potential impact of antipsychotic agents. *Psychoneuroendocrinology* **28** (Suppl. 2), 97–108.

Nakamura, Y., Koh, M., Miyoshi, E., *et al.* (2004) High prevalence of the hepatitis C virus infection among the inpatients of schizophrenia and psychoactive substance abuse in Japan. *Prog. Neuropsychopharmacol. Biol. Psychiatry* **28**, 591–597.

Nakane, Y., Ohta, Y. (1986) The example of linkage with a cancer register. In *Psychiatric Case Registers in Public Health*, eds. G. H. Ten Horn, R. Giel, W. H. Gulbinat. Amsterdam: Elsevier, pp. 240–245.

National Heart, Lung and Blood Institute (2001) *Definition of Hypertension.* Available online at www.ncbi.nlm.nih.gov/entrez/ query.fcgi?CMD=search&DB=pubmed

National Institutes of Health (2004) Consensus development conference on antipsychotic drugs and obesity and diabetes. *Diabetes Care* **27**, 596–601.

Negulici, E., Christodorescu, D. (1967) Paranoid schizophrenia and Klinefelter's syndrome. *Psychiatr. Neurol. (Basel)* **154**, 27–36.

Neimeier, R., Hauser, G. A., Keller, M., *et al.* (1959) [Pathological lactation.] *Schweiz. Med. Wochenschr.* **89**, 442–445.

Newcomer, J. W. (2005) Second-generation (atypical) antipsychotics and metabolic effects: a comprehensive literature review. *CNS Drugs* **19** (Suppl. 1), 1–93.

Newcomer, J. W., Haupt, D. W., Fucetola, R., *et al.* (2002) Abnormalities in glucose regulation during antipsychotic treatment of schizophrenia. *Arch. Gen. Psychiatry* **59**, 337–345.

Newman, S. C., Bland, R. C. (1991) Mortality in a cohort of patients with schizophrenia: a record linkage study. *Can. J. Psychiatry* **36**, 239–245.

Nicholson, G., Liebling, L. I., Hall, R. A. (1976) Thyroid dysfunction in female psychiatric patients. *Br. J. Psychiatry* **129**, 236–238.

Nilsson, E., Lichtenstein, P., Cnattingius, S., Murray, R. M., Hultman, C. M. (2002) Women with schizophrenia: pregnancy outcome and infant death among their offspring. *Schizophr. Res.* **58**, 221–229.

Nissen, H. A., Spencer, K. A. (1936) The psychogenic problem (endocrinal and metabolic) in chronic arthritis. *N. Engl. J. Med.* **21**, 567–581.

Nordenberg, J., Fenig, E., Landau, M., Weizman, R., Weizman, A. (1999) Effects of psychotropic drugs on cell proliferation and differentiation. *Biochem. Pharmacol.* **58**, 1229–1236.

Nyback, H., Wiesel, F. A., Berggren, B. M., Hindmarsh, T. (1982) Computed tomography of the brain in patients with acute psychosis and in healthy volunteers. *Acta Psychiatr. Scand.* **65**, 403–414.

O'Keane, V., Meaney, A. M. (2005) Antipsychotic drugs: a new risk factor for osteoporosis in young women with schizophrenia? *J. Clin. Psychopharmacol.* **25**, 26–31.

Ohta, Y., Nakane, Y., Mine, M., *et al.* (1988) The epidemiological study of physical morbidity in schizophrenics. 2. Association between schizophrenia and incidence of tuberculosis. *Jpn. J. Psychiatry Neurol.* **42**, 41–47.

Oken, R. J., Schulzer, M. (1999) At issue: schizophrenia and rheumatoid arthritis – the negative association revisited. *Schizophr. Bull.* **25**, 625–638.

Okura, M., Morii, S. (1986) Polydipsia, polyuria and water intoxication observed in psychiatric inpatients. *Tokushima J. Exp. Med.* **33**, 1–5.

Osborn, D. P., King, M. B., Nazareth, I. (2003) Participation in screening for cardiovascular risk by people with schizophrenia or similar mental illnesses: cross sectional study in general practice. *Br. Med. J.* **326**, 1122–1123.

Ostbye, T., Curtis, L. H., Masselink, L. E., *et al.* (2005) Atypical antipsychotic drugs and diabetes mellitus in a large outpatient population: a retrospective cohort study. *Pharmacoepidemiol. Drug Saf.* **14**, 407–415.

Osterberg, E. (1978) Schizophrenia and rheumatic disease: a study on the concurrence of inflammatory joint diseases and a review of 58 case-records. *Acta Psychiatr. Scand.* **58**, 339–359.

Osterlind, A. (1990) Malignant melanoma in Denmark: occurrence and risk factors. *Acta Oncol.* **29**, 833–854.

Othman, S. S., Abdul, K. K., Hassan, J., *et al.* (1994) High prevalence of thyroid function test abnormalities in chronic schizophrenia. *Aust. N. Z. J. Psychiatry* **28**, 620–624.

Oxenstierna, G., Bergstrand, G., Bjerkenstedt, L., Sedvall, G., Wik, G. (1984) Evidence of disturbed CSF circulation and brain atrophy in cases of schizophrenic psychosis. *Br. J. Psychiatry* **144**, 654–661.

Paffenberger R. S., Steinmetz, C. H., Pooler, B. G., Hyde, R. T. (1961) The picture puzzle of the postpartum psychosis. *J. Chronic Dis.* **13**, 161–173.

Palmer, B. A., Pankratz, V. S., Bostwick, J. M. (2005) The lifetime risk of suicide in schizophrenia: a re-examination. *Arch. Gen. Psychiatry* **62**, 247–253.

Paton, C., Esop, R., Young, C., Taylor, D. (2004) Obesity, dyslipidaemias and smoking in an inpatient population treated with antipsychotic drugs. *Acta Psychiatr. Scand.* **110**, 299–305.

Peh, L. H., Devan, G. S., Eu, P. W. (1990) Water intoxication in psychiatric patients in Singapore. *Singapore Med. J.* **31**, 238–241.

Pelissolo, A. (1997) [Epidemiology of psychopathologic disorders in infectious diseases.] *Encephale* **23**, (Spec. No. 5), 3–8.

Perisic, V. N., Lopicic, Z., Kokai, G. (1990) Celiac disease and schizophrenia: family occurrence. *J. Pediatr. Gastroenterol. Nutr.* **11**, 279.

Perkins, D. O. (2003) Prolactin- and endocrine-related disorders in schizophrenia. In *Medical Illness and Schizophrenia*, eds. J. M. Meyer, H. A. Nasrallah. Washington, DC: American Psychiatric Publishing, pp. 215–232.

Pilkington, T. L. (1956) The coincidence of rheumatoid arthritis and schizophrenia. *J. Nerv. Ment. Dis.* **124**, 604–606.

Preti, A., Cardascia, L., Zen, T., *et al.* (2000) Risk for obstetric complications and schizophrenia. *Psychiatr. Res.* **96**, 127–139.

Primatesta, P., Hirani, V. (1999) *Health Survey for England: The Health of Minority Ethnic Groups.* 1999. London: Department of Health. http://www.official-documents.co.uk. 2007.

Prohovnik, I., Dwork, A. J., Kaufman, M. A. Willson, N. (1993) Alzheimer-type neuropathology in elderly schizophrenia patients. *Schizophr. Bull.* **19**, 805–816.

Pryce, I. G., Edwards, H. (1966) Persistent oral dyskinesia in female mental hospital patients. *Br. J. Psychiatry* **112**, 983–987.

Py, O., Mathieu, P. (1960) [Galactorrhea and disorders of the menstrual cycle in the course of neuroleptic treatments.] *Presse Med.* **68**, 765–766.

Qin, P., Xu, H., Laursen, T. M., Vestergaard, M., Mortensen, P. B. (2005) Risk for schizophrenia and schizophrenia-like psychosis among patients with epilepsy: population-based cohort study. *Br. Med. J.* **331**, 23.

Ragins, N., Schachter, J., Elmer, E., *et al.* (1975) Infants and children at risk for schizophrenia: environmental and developmental observations. *J. Am. Acad. Child Psychiatry* **14**, 150–177.

Ramsay, R. A., Ananth, J., Engelsmann, F., *et al.* (1982) Schizophrenia and psychosomatic illness. *J. Psychosom. Res.* **26**, 33–42.

Ravichand, D. M., Sheshayamma, V., Lakshmi Kameshwari, V., Chakradhar, T. (2005) Thyroid hormones and antithyroid drugs. *Calicut Med. J.* **3**, e3.

Ray, W. A., Meredith, S., Thapa, P. B., *et al.* (2001) Antipsychotics and the risk of sudden cardiac death. *Arch. Gen. Psychiatry* **58**, 1161–1167.

Regenold, W. T., Thapar, R. K., Marano, C., Gavirneni, S., Kondapavuluru, P. V. (2002) Increased prevalence of type 2 diabetes mellitus among psychiatric inpatients with bipolar I affective and schizoaffective disorders independent of psychotropic drug use. *J. Affect. Disord.* **70**, 19–26.

Reilly, J. G., Ayis, S. A., Ferrier, I. N., Jones, S. J., Thomas, S. H. (2000) QTc-interval abnormalities and psychotropic drug therapy in psychiatric patients. *Lancet* **355**, 1048–1052.

Rieder, R. O., Rosenthal, D., Wender, P., Blumenthal, H. (1975) The offspring of schizophrenics. 1. Fetal and neonatal deaths. *Arch. Gen. Psychiatry* **32**, 200–211.

Rieder, R. O., Broman, S. H., Rosenthal, D. (1977) The offspring of schizophrenics. 2. Perinatal factors and IQ. *Arch. Gen. Psychiatry* **34**, 789–799.

Riggs, A. T., Dysken, M. W., Kim, S. W., Opsahl, J. A. (1991) A review of disorders of water homeostasis in psychiatric patients. *Psychosomatics* **32**, 133–148.

Rimon, R., Halonen, P., Puhakka, P., *et al.* (1979) Immunoglobulin G antibodies to herpes simplex type 1 virus detected by radioimmunoassay in serum and cerebrospinal fluid of patients with schizophrenia. *J. Clin. Psychiatry* **40**, 241–243.

Riscalla, L. M. (1980) Blindness and schizophrenia. *Med. Hypotheses* **6**, 1327–1328.

Robins, A. H. (1972) Phenothiazine melanosis in schizophrenic patients. *Psychopharmacologia* **27**, 327–342.

Roca, R. P., Blackman, M. R., Ackerley, M. B., Harman, S. M., Gregerman, R. I. (1990) Thyroid hormone elevations during acute psychiatric illness: relationship to severity and distinction from hyperthyroidism. *Endocr. Res.* **16**, 415–447.

Rodgers-Johnson, P. E., Hickling, F. W., Irons, A., *et al.* (1996) Retroviruses and schizophrenia in Jamaica. *Mol. Chem. Neuropathol.* **28**, 237–243.

Rose, D. P., Pruitt, B. T. (1981) Plasma prolactin levels in patients with breast cancer. *Cancer* **48**, 2687–2691.

Rosenberg, S. D., Goodman, L. A., Osher, F. C., *et al.* (2001) Prevalence of HIV, hepatitis B, and hepatitis C in people with severe mental illness. *Am. J. Public Health* **91**, 31–37.

Rosenthal, S. H., Porter, K. A., Coffey, B. (1990) Pain insensitivity in schizophrenia: case report and review of the literature. *Gen. Hosp. Psychiatry* **12**, 319–322.

Ross, W. D., Hay, J., McDowall, M. F. (1950) The association of certain vegetative disturbances with various psychoses. *Psychosom. Med.* **12**, 170–183.

Rothermich, N. O., Philips, V. K. (1963) Rheumatoid arthritis in criminal and mentally ill populations. *Arthritis Rheum.* **6**, 639–640.

Rotkin, I. D. (1977) Studies in the epidemiology of prostatic cancer: expanded sampling. *Cancer Treat. Rep.* **61**, 173–180.

Ruigomez, A., Garcia Rodriguez, L. A., Dev, V. J., Arellano, F., Raniwala, J. (2000) Are schizophrenia or antipsychotic drugs a risk factor for cataracts? *Epidemiology* **11**, 620–623.

Rwegellara, G. G. C., Mambwe, C. C. (1977) Psychiatric status and disorders of thyroid-function. 1. Prevalence of goiter in a group of psychiatric patients. *Med. J. Zambia* **11**, 78–83.

Ryan, M. C., Collins, P., Thakore, J. H. (2003) Impaired fasting glucose tolerance in first-episode, drug-naive patients with schizophrenia. *Am. J. Psychiatry* **160**, 284–289.

Ryan, W. G., Roddam, R. F., Grizzle, W. E. (1994) Thyroid function screening in newly admitted psychiatric inpatients. *Ann. Clin. Psychiatry* **6**, 7–12.

Rybakowski, J., Romanski, B., Dabkowska, M., Grabowski, P., Krymer, A. (1992) Allergic skin reactions in schizophrenia and affective disorders. *Biol. Psychiatry* **31**, 1181–1182.

Saari, K. M., Jokelainen, J., Veijola, J., *et al.* (2004) Serum lipids in schizophrenia and other functional psychoses: a general population northern Finland 1966 birth cohort survey. *Acta Psychiatr. Scand.* **110**, 279–285.

Saari, K. M., Lindeman, S. M., Viilo, K. M., *et al.* (2005) A 4-fold risk of metabolic syndrome in patients with schizophrenia: the Northern Finland 1966 Birth Cohort study. *J. Clin. Psychiatry* **66**, 559–563.

Sachdev, P. S. (1998) Schizophrenia-like psychosis and epilepsy: the status of the association. *Am. J. Psychiatry* **155**, 325–336.

Sachdev, P. S. (2000) The current status of tardive dyskinesia. *Aust. N. Z. J. Psychiatry* **34**, 355–369.

Sacker, A., Done, D. J., Crow, T. J. (1996) Obstetric complications in children born to parents with schizophrenia: a meta-analysis of case-control studies. *Psychol. Med.* **26**, 279–287.

Sacks, M. H., Dermatis, H., Looser-Ott, S., Burton, W., Perry, S. (1992) Undetected HIV infection among acutely ill psychiatric inpatients. *Am. J. Psychiatry* **149**, 544–545.

Sacks, M. H., Silberstein, C., Weiler, P., Perry, S. (1990) HIV-related risk factors in acute psychiatric inpatients. *Hosp. Commun. Psychiatry* **41**, 449–451.

Said, W. M., Saleh, R., Jumaian, N. (2001) Prevalence of hepatitis B virus among chronic schizophrenia patients. *East Mediterr. Health J.* **7**, 526–530.

Sameroff, A. J., Zax, M. (1973) Perinatal characteristics of the offspring of schizophrenic women. *J. Nerv. Ment. Dis.* **157**, 191–199.

Sandison, R. A., Whitelaw, E., Currie, J. D. (1960) Clinical trials with melleril (TP21) in the treatment of schizophrenia: *a two-year study. J. Ment. Sci.* **106**, 732–741.

Sartorius, N., Schulze, H. (eds.) (2005) *A Report of a Global Programme of the World Psychiatric Association*, eds. N. Sartorius, H. Schulze. Cambridge, UK: Cambridge University Press.

Schetlen, A. E. (1931) Malignant tumors in the institutionalized psychotic population. *Arch. Neurol. Psychiatry* **66**, 145–155.

Schneider, K. (1959) *Clinical Psychopathology*. New York: Grune & Stratton.

Schubert, E. W., McNeil, T. F. (2004) Prospective study of neurological abnormalities in offspring of women with psychosis: birth to adulthood. *Am. J. Psychiatry* **161**, 1030–1037.

Schubert, E. W., Blennow, G., McNeil, T. F. (1996) Wakefulness and arousal in neonates born to women with schizophrenia: diminished arousal and its association with neurological deviations. *Schizophr. Res.* **22**, 49–59.

Schwalb, H. (1975) [Risk factors of coronary heart diseases in hospitalized psychic patients.] *Munch. Med. Wochenschr.* **117**, 1181–1188.

Schwalb, H., van Eimeren, W., Friedrich, H. V. (1976) [The risk of heart disease in various psychiatric diseases.] *Z. Kardiol.* **65**, 1115–1123.

Schwartz-Watts, D., Montgomery, L. D., Morgan, D. W. (1995) Seroprevalence of human immunodeficiency virus among inpatient pretrial detainees. *Bull. Am. Acad. Psychiatr. Law* **23**, 285–288.

Secreto, G., Recchione, C., Cavalleri, A., Miraglia, M., Dati, V. (1983) Circulating levels of testosterone, 17 beta-oestradiol, luteinising hormone and prolactin in postmenopausal breast cancer patients. *Br. J. Cancer* **47**, 269–275.

Seeman, M. V., Lang, M., Rector, N. (1990) Chronic schizophrenia: a risk factor for HIV? *Can. J. Psychiatry* **35**, 765–768.

Sewell, D. D. (1996) Schizophrenia and HIV. *Schizophr. Bull.* **22**, 465–473.

Shader, R. I., Grinspoon, L. (1970) The effect of social feedback on chronic schizophrenic patients. *Compr. Psychiatry* **11**, 196–199.

Shah, P. J., Greenberg, W. M. (1992) Polydipsia with hyponatremia in a state hospital population. *Hosp. Commun. Psychiatry* **43**, 509–511.

Shinmoto, M., Kawarabayashi, T., Sugimori, H., *et al.* (1989) [The obstetric prognosis and neonatal outcome of pregnant women with psychiatric disorders.] *Nippon Sanka Fujinka Gakkai Zasshi* **41**, 1965–1971.

Sibai, B. M., Gordon, T., Thom, E., *et al.* (1995) Risk factors for preeclampsia in healthy nulliparous women: a prospective multicenter study – The National Institute of Child Health and Human Development Network of Maternal–Fetal Medicine Units. *Am. J. Obstet. Gynecol.* **172**, 642–648.

Sicree, R., Shaw, J., Zimmet, P. (2003) The global burden of diabetes. In *Diabetes Atlas*, ed D. Gan. Brussels: International Diabetes Federation, pp. 15–71.

Silberstein, C., Galanter, M., Marmor, M., *et al.* (1994) HIV-1 among inner city dually diagnosed inpatients. *Am. J. Drug Alcohol Abuse* **20**, 101–113.

Silver, H., Kogan, H., Zlotogorski, D. (1990) Postural hypotension in chronically medicated schizophrenics. *J. Clin. Psychiatry* **51**, 459–462.

Silverstone, T., Smith, G., Goodall, E. (1988) Prevalence of obesity in patients receiving depot antipsychotics. *Br. J. Psychiatry* **153**, 214–217.

Sim, K., Chong, S. A., Chan, Y. H., Lum, W. M. (2002) Thyroid dysfunction in chronic schizophrenia within a state psychiatric hospital. *Ann. Acad. Med. Singapore* **31**, 641–644.

Singh, M. K., Giles, L. L., Nasrallah, H. A. (2006) Pain insensitivity in schizophrenia: trait or state marker? *J. Psychiatr. Pract.* **12**, 90–102.

Singh, M. M., Kay, S. R. (1976) Wheat gluten as a pathogenic factor in schizophrenia. *Science* **191**, 401–402.

Siscovick, D. S., Raghunathan, T. E., Psaty, B. M., *et al.* (1994) Diuretic therapy for hypertension and the risk of primary cardiac arrest. *N. Engl. J. Med.* **330**, 1852–1857.

Sleeper, F. H. (1935) Investigation of polyuria in schizophrenia. *Am. J. Psychiatry* **91**, 1019–1031.

Smith, S. M., O'Keane, V., Murray, R. (2002) Sexual dysfunction in patients taking conventional antipsychotic medication. *Br. J. Psychiatry* **181**, 49–55.

Sobel, D. E. (1961) Children of schizophrenic patients: preliminary observations on early development. *Am. J. Psychiatry* **118**, 512–517.

Spector, T. D. (1990) Rheumatoid arthritis. *Rheum. Dis. Clin. North Am.* **16**, 513–537.

Spratt, D. I., Pont, A., Miller, M. B., *et al.* (1982) Hyperthyroxinemia in patients with acute psychiatric disorders. *Am. J. Med.* **73**, 41–48.

Stanley, H. L. Schmitt, B. P., Poses, R. M., Deiss, W. P. (1991) Does hypogonadism contribute to the occurrence of a minimal trauma hip tracture in elderly men? *J. Am. Geriatr. Soc.* **39**, 766–771.

Steiner, I., Abramsky, O. (1989) Autoimmune diseases of the neuroimmune system and mental disease. *Immunol. Ser.* **45**, 491–511.

Steinert, T., Wolfersdorf, M., Thoma, H., Marpert, M. (1996) [Does long-term hospitalization modify cardiovascular morbidity in schizophrenic patients?] *Fortschr. Neurol. Psychiatr.* **64**, 212–220.

Stevens, F. M., Lloyd, R. S., Geraghty, S. M., *et al.* (1977) Schizophrenia and coeliac disease: the nature of the relationship. *Psychol. Med.* **7**, 259–263.

Stewart, D. L., Zuckerman, C. J., Ingle, J. M. (1994) HIV seroprevalence in a chronically mentally ill population. *J. Natl Med. Assoc.* **86**, 519–523.

Subramaniam, M., Chong, S. A., Pek, E. (2003) Diabetes mellitus and impaired glucose tolerance in patients with schizophrenia. *Can. J. Psychiatry* **48**, 345–347.

Sugerman, A. A., Southern, D. L., Curran, J. F. (1982) A study of antibody levels in alcoholic, depressive and schizophrenic patients. *Ann. Allergy* **48**, 166–171.

Susser, E., Valencia, E., Conover, S. (1993) Prevalence of HIV infection among psychiatric patients in a New York City men's shelter. *Am. J. Public Health* **83**, 568–570.

Sweetwood, H. L., Kripke, D. F., Grant, I., Yager, J., Gerst, M. S. (1976) Sleep disorder and psychobiological symptomatology in male psychiatric outpatients and male nonpatients. *Psychosom. Med.* **38**, 373–378.

Taieb, O., Baleyte, J. M., Mazet, P., Fillet, A. M. (2001) Borna disease virus and psychiatry. *Eur. Psychiatry* **16**, 3–10.

Takahashi, K. I., Shimizu, T., Sugita, T., (1998) Prevalence of sleep-related respiratory disorders in 101 schizophrenic inpatients. *Psychiatr. Clin. Neurosci.* **52**, 229–231.

Tang, W. K., Sun, F. C., Ungvari, G. S., O'Donnell, D. (2004) Oral health of psychiatric in-patients in Hong Kong. *Int. J. Soc. Psychiatry* **50**, 186–191.

Taylor, D. C. (2003) Schizophrenias and epilepsies: why? when? how? *Epilepsy Behav.* **4**, 474–482.

Taylor, S. (1984) Gilbert's syndrome as a cause of postoperative jaundice. *Anaesthesia* **39**, 1222–1224.

Templer, D. I., Cappelletty, G. G., Kauffman, I. (1988) Schizophrenia and multiple sclerosis: *distribution in Italy. Br. J. Psychiatry* **153**, 389–390.

Templer, D. I., Regier, M. W., Corgiat, M. D. (1985) Similar distribution of schizophrenia and multiple sclerosis. *J. Clin. Psychiatry* **46**, 73.

Terenius, L., Wahlstrom, A. (1978) Physiologic and clinical relevance of endorphins. In *Centrally Acting Peptides*, ed. J. Hughes Baltimore, MD: Baltimore University Park Press, pp. 161–178.

Test, M. A., Wallisch, L. S., Allness, D. J., Ripp, K. (1989) Substance abuse in young adults with schizophrenic disorders. *Schizophr. Bull.* **15**, 465–476.

Teunissen, C. E., de Vente, J., Steinbusch, H. W., De Bruijn, C. (2002) Biochemical markers related to Alzheimer's dementia in serum and cerebrospinal fluid. *Neurobiol. Aging* **23**, 485–508.

Thakore, J. H., Mann, J. N., Vlahos, I., Martin, A., Reznek, R. (2002) Increased visceral fat distribution in drug-naive and drug-free patients with schizophrenia. *Int. J. Obes. Relat Metab. Disord.* **26**, 137–141.

Theisen, F. M., Linden, A., Geller, F., *et al.* (2001) Prevalence of obesity in adolescent and young adult patients with and without schizophrenia and in relationship to antipsychotic medication. *J. Psychiatr. Res.* **35**, 339–345.

Thomas, A., Lavrentzou, E., Karouzos, C., Kontis, C. (1996) Factors which influence the oral condition of chronic schizophrenia patients. *Spec. Care Dentist* **16**, 84–86.

Tishler, P. V., Woodward, B., O'Connor, J., *et al.* (1985) High prevalence of intermittent acute porphyria in a psychiatric patient population. *Am. J. Psychiatry* **142**, 1430–1436.

Torrey, E. F. (1979) Headaches after lumbar puncture and insensitivity to pain in psychiatric patients. *N. Engl. J. Med.* **301**, 110.

Torrey, E. F. (1997) *Out of the Shadows: Confronting America's Mental Illness Crisis.* New York: John Wiley.

Torrey, E. F., Peterson, M. R. (1973) Slow and latent viruses in schizophrenia. *Lancet* **ii**, 22–24.

Torrey, E. F., Yolken, R. H. (2001) The schizophrenia–rheumatoid arthritis connection: infectious, immune, or both? *Brain Behav. Immun.* **15**, 401–410.

Torrey, E. F., Yolken, R. H. (2003) *Toxoplasma gondii* and schizophrenia. *Emerg. Infect. Dis.* **9**, 1375–1380.

Trevathan, R. D., Tatum, J. C. (1954) Rarity of occurrence of psychosis and rheumatoid arthritis in individual patients. *J. Nerv. Ment. Dis.* **120**, 83–84.

Tsuang, M. T., Fleming, J. A., Simpson, J. C. (1999) Suicide and schizophrenia. In *The Harvard Medical School Guide to Suicide Assessment and Intervention*, ed. D. G. Jacobs. San Francisco, CA: Jossey-Bass, pp. 287–299

Turkington, R. W. (1972) Prolactin secretion in patients treated with various drugs: phenothiazines, tricyclic antidepressants, reserpine, and methyldopa. *Arch. Intern. Med.* **130**, 349–354.

Ural, S. (2004) What is the Apgar score? Available online at www.kidshealth.org/ parent/newborn/first_days/apgar.html

Varsamis, J., Adamson, J. D. (1976) Somatic symptoms in schizophrenia. *Can. Psychiatr. Assoc. J.* **21**, 1–6.

Velasco, E., Machuca, G., Martinez-Sahuquillo, A., *et al.* (1997) Dental health among institutionalized psychiatric patients in Spain. *Spec. Care Dentist* **17**, 203–206.

Velasco-Ortega, E., Monsalve-Guil, L., Velasco-Ponferrada, C., Medel-Soteras, R., Segura-Egea, J. J. (2005) Temporomandibular disorders among schizophrenic patients: a case-control study. *Med. Oral Patol. Oral Cir. Bucal.* **10**, 315–322.

Vieweg, W. V., David, J. J., Glick, J. L., *et al.* (1986) Polyuria among patients with psychosis. *Schizophr. Bull.* **12**, 739–743.

Vieweg, W. V., David, J. J., Rowe, W. T., *et al.* (1985) Death from self-induced water intoxication among patients with schizophrenic disorders. *J. Nerv. Ment. Dis.* **173**, 161–165.

Viskum, K. (1975) Mind and ulcer. *Acta Psychiatr. Scand.* **51**, 182–200.

Volavka, J., Convit, A., Czobor, P., *et al.* (1991) HIV seroprevalence and risk behaviors in psychiatric inpatients. *Psychiatr. Res.* **39**, 109–114.

Wainberg, M. L., Cournos, F., McKinnon, K., Berkman, A. (2003) HIV and hepatitis C in patients with schizophrenia. In *Medical Illness and Schizophrenia*, eds. J. M. Meyer, H. A. Nasrallah. Washington, DC: American Psychiatric Publishing, pp. 115–140.

Warner, J. P., Barnes, T. R., Henry, J. A. (1996) Electrocardiographic changes in patients receiving neuroleptic medication. *Acta Psychiatr. Scand.* **93**, 311–313.

Watson, G. D., Chandarana, P. C., Merskey, H. (1981) Relationships between pain and schizophrenia. *Br. J. Psychiatry* **138**, 33–36.

Webb, R., Abel, K., Pickles, A., Appleby, L. (2005) Mortality in offspring of parents with psychotic disorders: a critical review and meta-analysis. *Am. J. Psychiatry* **162**, 1045–1056.

Weinberg, A. D., Katzell, T. D. (1977) Thyroid and adrenal function among psychiatric patients. *Lancet* **i**, 1104–1105.

Weinreb, M., Kraus, V., Krausova, J., Hudcova, T. (1978) Negligible hepatotoxicity of chlorpromazine in long-term therapy. *Acta. Nerv. Super. (Praha)* **20**, 280–281.

Wesselmann, U., Windgassen, K. (1995) Galactorrhea: subjective response by schizophrenic patients. *Acta Psychiatr. Scand.* **91**, 152–155.

Wetterling, T., Pest, S., Mussigbrodt, H., Weber, B. (2004) [Bodyweight in inpatients with schizophrenia.] *Psychiatr. Prax.* **31**, 250–254.

White, K. E., Cummings, J. L. (1996) Schizophrenia and Alzheimer's disease: clinical and pathophysiologic analogies. *Compr. Psychiatry* **37**, 188–195.

Wieck, A., Haddad, P. M. (2003) Antipsychotic-induced hyperprolactinaemia in women: pathophysiology, severity and consequences – selective literature review. *Br. J. Psychiatry* **182**, 199–204.

Wiedorn, W. S. (1954) Toxemia of pregnancy and schizophrenia. *J. Nerv. Ment. Dis.* **120**, 1–9.

Windgassen, K., Wesselmann, U., Schulze, M. H. (1996) Galactorrhea and hyperprolactinemia in schizophrenic patients on neuroleptics: frequency and etiology. *Neuropsychobiology* **33**, 142–146.

Winkelman, J. W. (2001) Schizophrenia, obesity, and obstructive sleep apnea. *J. Clin. Psychiatry* **62**, 8–11.

Wolff, A. L., O'Driscoll, G. A. (1999) Motor deficits and schizophrenia: the evidence from neuroleptic-naive patients and populations at risk. *J. Psychiatr. Neurosci.* **24**, 304–314.

World Health Organization (1992) *International Statistical Classification of Diseases and Related Health Problems*, 10th revn. Geneva: World Health Organization.

World Health Organization (1999) *Report of a WHO Consultation: Definition, Diagnosis and Classification of Diabetes Mellitus and its Complications. Part I:Diagnosis and Classification of Diabetes Mellitus.* Geneva: World Health Organization.

World Health Organization (2001) *World Health Report 2001: Mental Health – New Understanding, New Hope.* Geneva: World Health Organization.

World Health Organization (2004) *HIV and AIDS Statistics and Features, End of 2002 and 2004.* Available online at www.unaids.org/wad2004/EPIupdate2004_html_en/Epi04_12_en.htm#P227_67386

Wrede, G., Mednick, S. A., Huttunen, M. O., Nilsson, C. G. (1980) Pregnancy and delivery complications in the births of an unselected series of Finnish children with schizophrenic mothers. *Acta Psychiatr. Scand.* **62**, 369–381.

Yase, Y., Matsumoto, N., Azuma, K., Nakai, Y., Shiraki, H. (1972) Amyotrophic lateral sclerosis: association with schizophrenic symptoms and showing Alzheimer's tangles. *Arch. Neurol.* **27**, 118–128.

Young, T., Palta, M., Dempsey, J., *et al.* (1993) The occurrence of sleep-disordered breathing among middle-aged adults. *N. Engl. J. Med.* **328**, 1230–1235.

Zamperetti, M., Goldwurm, G. F., Abbate, E., *et al.* (1990) Attempted suicide and HIV infection: epidemiological aspects in a psychiatric ward. *International Conference on AIDS, San Francisco, CA.*

Zaridze, D. G., Boyle, P. (1987) Cancer of the prostate: epidemiology and aetiology. *Br. J. Urol.* **59**, 493–502.

Zax, M., Sameroff, A. J., Babigian, H. M. (1977) Birth outcomes in the offspring of mentally disordered women. *Am. J. Orthopsychiatry* **47**, 218–230.

Zeenreich, A., Gochstein, B., Grinshpoon, A., *et al.* (1998) [Recurrent tuberculosis in a psychiatric hospital: recurrent outbreaks during 1987–1996.] *Harefuah* **134**, 168–172, 248, 247.

Zhang-Wong, J. H., Seeman, M. V. (2002) Antipsychotic drugs, menstrual regularity and osteoporosis risk. *Arch. Women Ment. Health* **5**, 93–98.

Zimmet, P. (2005) Epidemiology of diabetes mellitus and associated cardiovascular risk factors: focus on human immunodeficiency virus and psychiatric disorders. *Am. J. Med.* **118** (Suppl. 2), 3S-8S.

Zito, J. M., Sofair, J. B., Jaeger, J. (1990) Self-reported neuroendocrine effects of antipsychotics in women: a pilot study. *Drug Intell. Clin. Pharmacy* **24**, 176–180.

Index

Note: page numbers in *italics* refer to tables